I0104542

I Left My Thighs in San Francisco

How You Can Use A New Time-Saving System
for Weight Loss,
Exercise, More Energy, and
Being Happy WHILE You Drop Weight

Tom Marcoux

Executive Coach

Spoken Word Strategist

TFG Thought Leader

Speaker-Author of 27 books

Blogger, BeHeardandBeTrusted.com

A QuickBreakthrough Publishing Edition

Copyright © 2015 Tom Marcoux Media, LLC
ISBN: 0692459510
ISBN-13: 978-0692459515
All rights reserved. No part of this book may be reproduced or transmitted in any form by any means electronic or mechanical, including photocopying, recording or by any information storage and retrieval system without written permission from the publisher.

QuickBreakthrough Publishing is an imprint of Tom Marcoux Media, LLC. More copies are available from the publisher, Tom Marcoux Media, LLC. Please call (415) 572-6609 or write TomSuperCoach@gmail.com

or visit www.TomSuperCoach.com

or Tom's blog: www.BeHeardandBeTrusted.com

This book was developed and written with care. Names and details were modified to respect privacy.

Disclaimer: The author and publisher acknowledge that each person's situation is unique, and that readers have full responsibility to seek consultations with health, financial, spiritual and legal professionals. The author and publisher make no representations or warranties of any kind, and the author and publisher shall not be liable for any special, consequential or exemplary damages resulting, in whole or in part, from the reader's use of, or reliance upon, this material.:

Other Books by Tom Marcoux:
- Be Heard and Be Trusted: How to Get What You Want
- Nothing Can Stop You This Year!
- Reduce Clutter, Enlarge Your Life
- Darkest Secrets of Persuasion and Seduction Masters
- Darkest Secrets of Charisma
- Darkest Secrets of Negotiation Masters
- Darkest Secrets of the Film and Television Industry Every Actor Should Know
- Darkest Secrets of Making a Pitch to the Film and Television Industry
- Darkest Secrets of Film Directing
- Truth No One Will Tell You

Praise for *I Left My Thighs in San Francisco* and Tom Marcoux:

• "In *I Left My Thighs in San Francisco*, you learn ways to feel good, look great, and use time-saving secrets for more personal energy!"
– Dr. JoAnn Dahlkoetter, author, *Your Performing Edge* and Coach to CEOs and Olympic Gold Medalists
• "Tom Marcoux has distinguished himself as a coach, speaker and self-help author. His books combine his own philosophy and teachings, as well as those of other success experts, in a highly readable and relatable manner." – Danek S. Kaus, co-author of *Power Persuasion*

Praise for Tom Marcoux's Other Work:
• "In Tom Marcoux's *Now You See Me*, the powerful and easy-to-use ideas can make a big difference in your business and your personal relationships." – Allen Klein, author of *You Can't Ruin My Day*
• "Marcoux's book *10 Seconds to Wealth* focuses on how each of us have divine gifts that we need to understand and use to be our best when the crucial '10 seconds' occur.... He identifies the divine gifts and shares how these gifts can help us create what we want in our lives, and the wealth we want." – Linda Finkle, author of *Finding The Fork In The Road: The Art of Maximizing the Potential of Business Partnerships*
• "In *Darkest Secrets of Persuasion and Seduction Masters: How to Protect Yourself and Turn the Power to Good,* learn useful countermeasures to protect you from being darkly manipulated."
– David Barron, co-author, *Power Persuasion*
• "In *Be Heard and Be Trusted*, Tom's advice on how to remain true to yourself and establish authentic rapport with clients is both insightful and reality based. He [shows how] to establish oneself as a credible expert."
- Arthur P. Ciaramicoli, Ed.D., Ph.D., author *The Curse of the Capable*
• "In *Reduce Clutter, Enlarge Your Life*, Marcoux will help you get rid of the physical and mental clutter occupying precious space in your life. You'll reclaim wasted energy, lower your stress, and find time for new opportunities." – Laura Stack, author of *Execution IS the Strategy*

Visit Tom's blog: www.BeHeardandBeTrusted.com

Tom Marcoux

CONTENTS

DEDICATION AND ACKNOWLEDGEMENTS

This book is dedicated to the terrific book and film consultant, and author Johanna E. Mac Leod. It is also dedicated to the other team members. Thanks to Barry Adamson II for editing. Thanks to David MacDowell Blue for editing of one section.

Thanks to guest authors Mark Sanborn, Jeanna Gabellini, Noah St. John, C.J. Hayden, Jeff Davidson, Patricia Fripp, Randy Gage, Willie Jolley, Rebecca Morgan, Dr. Elayne Savage, Craig Harrison, Lois Creamer, Pat Baldridge Chris Shelton, Linda Finkle and Coco of Light By Coco. [Their articles remain with their original copyright and are included in this book by their permission.]

Thank you to Judita Bacinskaite for rendering the front cover of this book. Thanks to Johanna E. MacLeod for the back cover. Thanks to my father, Al Marcoux, for his concern and efforts for me. Thanks to my mother, Sumiyo Marcoux, a kind, generous soul. Thank you to Higher Power. Thanks to our readers, audiences, clients, my graduate/college students and my team members of Tom Marcoux Media, LLC. The best to you.

Book One:
Discover How You Can Be Happy
WHILE You Lose Weight

My dear friend Cynthia climbed up the ten steps to get on the plane and found she was out of breath. Then she sat in the seat near me and grunted. She was so big that the arm rests of her seat were going to *squeeze* her for the whole flight.

Hearing her grunt, I recalled that her diabetic mother also grunted, in pain because her feet hurt with each step.

Cynthia was only 40 at the time, but she looked 60. A disabled 60.

It hurt seeing my friend endure so much pain.

Often, after I give a speech, people ask me, "Do you have a book on weight loss?"

Up until now, I've had to say, "No."

But now you have this book in your hands, so the answer has become *yes*.

Longing to be of service to Cynthia and people in her situation, I realized that *a different type of weight loss book* was called for. Why? **I am realistic. Many of us are *not* going to devote three hours a day to exercise. And we are *not* going to eat perfectly.**

I don't You don't. I know because you're reading these words.

You don't have to eat perfectly or exercise three hours a day. You can make excellent progress to drop extra weight and to look and feel better!

As a speaker and personal coach for over two decades, I continue helping people make big dreams come true.

Now, I'm here, through this book, **to help you to move forward with your drop-weight plans—and in realistic ways.**

Can you imagine a Different Kind of Book for Weight Loss?

I did imagine it; and *this book is for you!*

This is NOT a book of exercises and recipes.

You might wonder about the title *I Left My Thighs in San Francisco.* It's true. I was born and raised in San Francisco as a chubby kid. I learned how to integrate exercise into my daily life.

I've learned in my own life and with clients that **your *Drop-Weight Plan* needs to be supported by 3 Elements.**

A *Drop-Weight Plan* is a realistic process that provides methods for you to integrate new actions into your already busy life. New actions include exercise and healthy diet choices.

By the way, many people give up on New Years Resolutions because they do *not* use the 3 Elements.

To help everyone, including me, remember *the 3 Elements* of a good Drop-Weight Plan easily, I use the word S.E.E.:

S – strategize to fit your busy life

E – energize through Happy Moments

E – excel with More Time

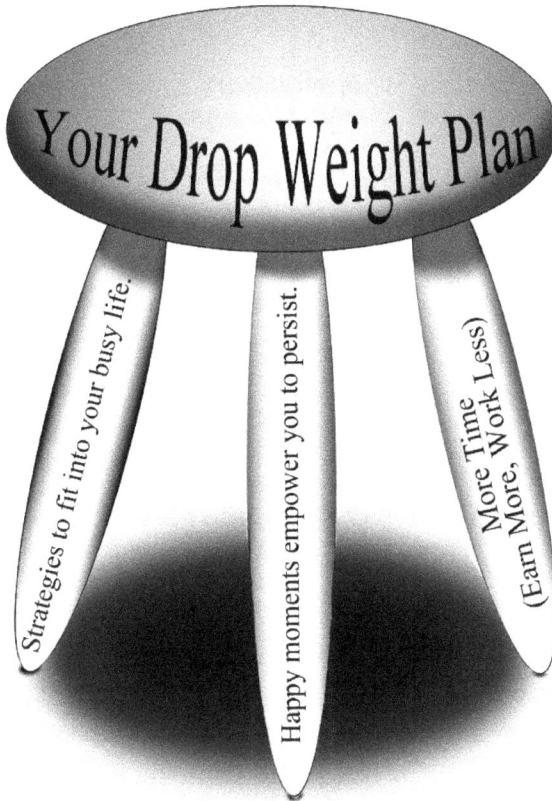

©Tom Marcoux Media, LLC

Image 1.1 See the support?

Here is *The Principle of this book:* **Dropping Weight is NOT done in a vacuum. The rest of your life needs to**

support your Drop-Weight Plan.

So this book includes three sections:

1) Strategize to fit your busy life
2) Energize through Happy Moments
   (Happy moments empower you to persist.)
3) Excel with More Time
   (Gain more time when you *Earn More, Work Less*)

How You Can Be Happy WHILE You Drop Weight

This book includes a whole section on *how to nurture your happiness WHILE you drop weight.*

I like the words "drop weight" instead of "lose weight." You're *not* losing weight; you are *not* losing anything. Instead you're releasing weight. I even prefer the words "get lighter."

Keeping with this positive approach, I refer to the process in this book as *the "Do NOT Torture Yourself System."*

Why is having happy moments each day important? You need personal energy to persist and to take care of yourself. Having happy moments each day truly increases your personal energy. Imagine that each person starts a new day with a pie of energy. Some people have a pie as big as a large pizza, and others only have a pie the size of a dinner mint. **Happy moments make a bigger pie of energy.** My clients can attest to that!

My client Angela said, "I find that when I make sure to have some happy moments, I can face my treadmill." In the beginning, Angela would walk briskly on her treadmill for 10 minutes and then take a break for tea. Then she got back on her treadmill for ten more minutes.

My client Shirley said, "I find that when I take a walk with my son the blocks go by, and I don't feel like I'm pushing myself."

I coach clients in ways to fit exercise into their busy lives. I live this process, too. For example, each day I aim to walk 10,000 steps and I integrate that goal in two ways. First, I have a daily walk with my sweetheart and we have a great conversation that nurtures our relationship. Second, I read while I walk on a treadmill.

A sidenote about the title "I Left My Thighs in San Francisco." Back on December 30, 2009, I thought of this title and registered the URL. In part, I'm sure the idea arose because, as I mentioned, I was born and raised a chubby kid in San Francisco. Taking karate classes and judo classes as a nine year old helped me get used to my growing body. In fact, I learned judo in a program run by the San Francisco Police Activities League. In college, I lifted weights and became trim and muscular. Yes, I did "leave my thighs in San Francisco"!

Now, several years later, I still do martial arts movements and I've added yoga to the mix.

Important Point: *This book is different from other books on weight loss.* I mean it! You're going to learn things beyond exercise tips and recipes. Get ready to fit in exercise and *make time* to truly persist with your Drop-Weight Plan.

Here are a just a few of the topics:
- Fit exercise in with "The Power of 10"
- Learn to Delegate Well So You Have More Time
- *Earn More* So You Can Cut Down Your Work Hours (gain time to exercise and rest well)

Let's begin:

Part One: Strategize to Fit Your Busy Life

20 Methods for Exercising, Eating Better and Fitting Weight-Dropping Activities into Your Busy Life:

We'll begin with the **P.O.W.E.R.** process:
P – Power-up "10"
O – organize Top Six Targets
W – work the strategy for exercise
E – engage the Trigger-Set Method
R – rig a "success system" and drop "perfectionism-pain"

1. Power-up "10"
To start developing your fitness, especially when you're busy, consider *"The Power of 10"* which I also call the *"Mighty Minimum."*

For example, when I was directing a feature film, the Power of 10 meant to me:
- 10 palm strikes
- 10 front kicks
- 10 side kicks
- 10 sit-ups
- 10 pushups
- 10 oblique sit-ups

Doing the above exercises might take only five minutes, and still, this process is working several major muscle groups.

The Power of 10 can be applied to weight training, too.

One does **10 lifting moves per arm** for a total of 20.
- 20 bicep curls

- 20 forward lifts for part of the shoulder
- 20 sideways lifts for another part of the shoulder
- 20 leaning over lifts for another part of the shoulder
- 20 triceps-related lifts
- 20 forearms-related lifts.

The above weight training can be done in five minutes or less.

CAUTION: Consult a doctor about your own fitness level when considering any exercise regimen.

The Power of 10 can apply to 10 minutes on the treadmill. The Big Benefit is that at 10 minutes, it often feels like "That was easy." This means that you won't dread tomorrow's 10 minutes on the treadmill.

The Power of 10 relates to what I call the *Mighty Minimum.* Imagine that you do a minimum of 10 sit-ups a day. That's 300 per month and 3,600 sit-ups per year—a real gain in core strength. In a way, we can say the minimum number of sit-ups makes you "mighty."

This reminds me of a quote from Joss Whedon's TV show *Firefly:* "We've done the impossible, and that makes us mighty."

A side note: One of my editors said that this "Power of 10" seems "too easy." I replied, "I'm looking for daily progress. I emphasize *better than zero.* After a good start, any individual can pursue expanding their exercise regimen in ways that apply to their individual needs."

2. Organize *Top Six Targets*

Just before you go to sleep, consider writing your *Top Six Targets*—the most important tasks for your next day. Each week, I write "weights" a few times as one of my Top Six Targets for the next day. With Top Six Targets, you identify what will make your day successful. Addressing audiences, I say, "2 for you, 2 for family, and 2 for work." This is a great method for prioritizing, and it gives you "marching orders" so you get into action faster the next day.

3. Work the strategy for exercise

Focus on *keep moving*. Research has shown that thinner people simply move more than heavier people. They walk up and down stairs, and even some twitch their foot when sitting. When I say "work the strategy for exercise," I mean work in exercise throughout the day. For example, during a break, I take the stairs when I'm on campus where I teach college students.

The strategy of "keep moving" works for entering your home to begin exercise so you step straight over to your treadmill.

One of my clients closes the door and (as she tells me) exercises in her underwear for "10 Terrific Minutes."

To get more out of her 10 minutes on the treadmill, she has the front of the treadmill raised so her session is all "walking uphill."

4. Engage the *Trigger-Set Method*

Everyday, you and I react to triggers. How? Imagine you like cookies and your family member leave them out on the living room table. Will you eat a cookie? Many people reply: "Probably." The real answer is often "Yes!"

What's the solution? Place the cookies into the cupboard where you cannot see them. This way the negative trigger of seeing the cookies does *not* happen.

Here's another strategy about triggers:

"Set the Positive Trigger when the situation is COOL –

So you automatically do the positive action when the situation is HOT."

For example, I have a positive trigger in my bedroom: a treadmill that is clear of anything on it.

With audiences, I often observe, "Do you have stationary bicycle? Yes—it's the most expensive towel rack."

So be strategic. Set up a positive trigger and avoid clogging it with towels!

5. Rig a "success system" and drop "perfectionism-pain"

We can effectively develop and use a *success system* when we identify what we most want and create an incremental way to achieve it.

Still, for many of us, a stumbling block is what I call *Perfectionism-Pain*—which often arises from *comparison.* If you compare yourself to professional athletes, actors, and actresses related to appearance, then such thoughts of trying to *compete* can send you into a downward, negative spiral. This creates real pain.

For the most part, this book is *not* designed for the professional athlete nor some young, genetically-gifted, stereotypically attractive person.

You might notice my choice of the above words.

For example, at this moment, I have gray hair at my temples. I am NOT trying to look younger than I am. Sure, I have footage of myself starring in a feature film when I was in my 20's. I don't watch it. *I own who I am today.*

In essence, I do NOT compete with my younger self.

My point is: *Drop Perfectionism-Pain.* Avoid trying to look perfect like a professional athlete or professional actor/actress.

Instead, pick your own goals to be a great version of *Yourself.*

I often say, "Don't compete, *connect.*"

Connect with your own heartfelt goals. *Many of us realize that we really want to be fit and healthy.* Also, for many of us, being healthy means dropping excess belly fat but we do not need six pack abs.

One of my friends, Joe, when he was a model achieved six pack abs. I asked him how he did it. "I eat soups," was his quick response.

So Joe was willing to pay the price for his six pack abs. After all, his appearance *was* his profession.

In this book, we're talking about *integrating* exercise into your busy life.

So what do we do when a "perfectionism thought" arises? Here are examples my clients have mentioned:

Perfectionism Thoughts:

- "Oh, look at her. She's got buns of steel. I've got buns of cellulite."
- "Oh, look at that guy. He could wear a Superman outfit. I could wear a whale outfit."

Perfectionism Thoughts are all about comparison. Shift your thoughts *to what you are doing for your health.*

The strategy is to shift from a Perfectionism Thought to what I call *"The Empowering Second Thought."* It really helps to condition yourself to have an instant, empowering response when a negative thought arises.

Stephen's pattern is this:

Perfectionism Thought: "Oh, look at that guy. He could wear a Superman outfit. I could wear a whale outfit."

Empowering Second Thought: "I'm making progress. I'm five pounds closer to my goal, and I am walking right now!"

Now, we'll continue building your Success System.

The Elements of a "Success System":

To set a habit takes more than 30 days. Why? Because once we get to the 30 day mark, many of us relax our vigilance and indulge in some diet-busting behavior. Some authors suggest that habit-building may take 40 days. In any case, we can use strategies to build our empowering habits. We'll use the C.A.N. process:

C – connects to your current activities

A – automatically-works

N – nurtures your feelings

Connects to your current activities. It helps to "attach" a new behavior to something you already naturally do. I read every day so a good plan is for me to read and walk on a treadmill. The added benefit is that reading makes the time go by pleasantly while I'm on the treadmill.

Automatically-works. By this I mean that you set up an automatic, positive behavior. Researchers talk about the benefits of positive habits. The idea is that you only make the decision once and then you automatically carry it out. For example, my sweetheart and I set up an *automatic behavior*. After dinner and the dishes are in the dish washing machine, she and I immediately leave for our evening walk and conversation. There is no hesitation. We do not make a new decision. We automatically take action.

Nurtures your feelings. We do so much just to get a good feeling. Why do people drink soda? It's an enjoyable experience. See if you can develop your exercise routine so that you enjoy some good experiences. I like talking with my sweetheart so it's great that we can combine our conversation with an evening walk.

For more about our feelings . . .

A Brief Discussion about Addiction

"I'm addicted to chocolate," my friend Anne said with enthusiasm. Is that true?

Dr. Michael F Roizen wrote: "When we talk about addiction circuitry, it comes down to these factors: a) If the behavior has a beneficial effect in the short term but adverse consequences in the long term, b) if the person develops a tolerance . . . and then needs more and more…, and c) if the person experiences symptoms of withdrawal…when he or she tries to stop doing the behavior."

For many of us the short term benefit is a rise in dopamine and endorphins (the feel-good substances in the body). Some of us get a rush of good feelings from a donut or ice cream. Our brain makes a connection: "I want to feel good so I'll get more donuts!"

To change our behavior is often more than a simple dropping of a bad habit. We often need to learn to replace the habit with something that helps us feel better.

Serena replaced a donut with an orange and dancing around (when at home alone) to her favorite invigorating music. She has strategically replaced eating a donut with another behavior that helps her feel good—and fast!

I often write about: **"Set the Positive Trigger when the situation is COOL—so you automatically take action when the situation is HOT."**

For Serena, the "hot" situation is arriving home after work. She's tired and she wants a treat. It takes well-considered strategy to replace reflexive-eating behaviors.

Other details about addiction (alcohol, drugs, etc.) are beyond the scope of this book.

Still it is valuable to examine your own behaviors and see if you appear to have some addictive patterns.

My point is that setting a Success System and being aware

of any perfectionism thoughts helps you stay consistent with your Drop-Weight Plan.

* * *

Our next six methods focus on **W.I.N.N.E.R.** You can feel like a winner when you keep moving and making incremental progress. What are you winning? You're winning against inertia. Every positive thing you do is *better than zero.*

W – work out what you really want
I – intensify the good trend
N – nurture daily fun
N – "neutralize" your state of being
E – escape the weight scale sometimes
R – repeat sessions (Power of 3 x 10)

1. Work out what you really want
Do you want to feel better? To live longer? To avoid certain diseases like diabetes?

When we're clear on what we *really* want, then we can do the most important things.

On the other hand, some of us wish for the "perfect body," but we do NOT really want to pay the required price for that six-pack abs or movie star buttocks.

Perhaps, you're considering having a more attractive body. What is something you feel you *Must Have*? Start there. For me, I must have good health. I must have lots of energy to devote to accomplishing my dreams. So that is my springboard to exercise and good nutrition.

What are your "must haves"?

2. Intensify the good trend

"I've dropped three pounds," my sweetheart told me yesterday. I replied, "Great! That's a good trend!"

The problem often arises that we discount or simply ignore a good outcome. Perhaps, we think that the gain is "too small."

To intensify a good trend is to *Celebrate Each Small Victory*. Did you drop one pound? Acknowledge it. Celebrate with a trusted friend. Have some fun together. Maybe take a walk together. Keep the good trend going.

3. Nurture daily fun

Have Some Fun Everyday—so you don't turn to food. Have you ever told yourself something like "I deserve ice cream today because I got the tax return done"?

Not having some form of fun on a daily basis makes you vulnerable to turning to food. How? You are likely to feel deprived on some level.

Some authors refer to the "inner child," that part of us that feels small, vulnerable and, wait for it, wants Some Fun!

The inner child is the source of your personal energy that you need for your Drop-Weight Plan. So pay attention to nurturing your inner child.

You need to identify an activity that is actually FUN. For example, for introverts some alone time/quiet time is most helpful for recharging.

I find it helpful to assemble a jigsaw puzzle while listening to stand up comedy on YouTube. Even just nine minutes provides uplifting energy to my day. If I miss some time for laughter, my day will feel off.

Now it's your turn.

What can give you some minutes of FUN today?

3. "Neutralize" your state of being

Sometimes we find that it's truly hard to shift out of a painful state of being. For example, one of my Facebook friends, Sarah, mentioned that her six year old, adorable cat died from complications during surgery.

I replied, "Oh! I grieve with you."

For Sarah, being asked to shift from grieving to a "happy state of being" may be asking too much.

Instead, we look to shift to a "neutral" state of being. This involves shifting to neutral thoughts and the present moment.

She might find attending a jazzercise class takes her mind off of her loss for sixty minutes.

Sarah then might say, "I'm okay. Not happy. But I'm okay."

4. Escape the weight scale sometimes

I remember a speaker saying, "Stay away from that thing (weight scale), it makes you cry!"

Weight Watchers does a weekly weigh-in. That's a good plan. For many of us, checking one's weight every day is too much of an emotional roller-coaster. Instead, we're looking for a weekly data-point that shows our positive trend.

Daily you move and focus on techniques that help your Drop-Weight Plan. For example, you can use a small bowl to reduce the size of your portions.

Additionally, if you weigh yourself once every seven days, you might call the other days "a vacation from the weight scale."

5. Repeat sessions (Power of 3 x 10)

Yesterday, I did three sessions of ten minutes each on my treadmill. Yes, I know that 30 minutes in a row might yield better results, but I'm still glad that my total time on the treadmill was 30 minutes for the day.

This strategy can be especially helpful when you're starting up or restarting an exercise program. You condition your body when you exercise for 10 minutes, then take a break, then exercise for ten more minutes. Over time, you adjust the Power of 3x10 to fit your needs and your schedule.

One of my clients, Andrea, has shifted up to 3 x 15 minutes. That's good! She has built upon her foundation of her Drop-Weight Plan.

* * *

Our next nine methods focus on L.I.G.H.T.E.N. U.P. as in "drop weight and lighten up."

L – locate your "Instant Feel Good HEALTHY" Action
I – ignite small disciplines
G – go for the spoonful not the bucket
H – Honor "Better than Zero"
T - take action with what you have
E – employ the "Power of Declaring"
N - Note and regulate your Comfort Food
U – use a pedometer
P – place the "Worst First" task

1. Locate your "Instant Feel Good HEALTHY" Action
The idea is to identify what helps you quickly feel better, but it's something that does NOT hurt you long term. I've asked a number of people as to what helps them feel better fast and many reply: "Chocolate" or "Diet Coke." Extra calories or caffeine can have harmful effects over the long

term.

On the other hand, we can choose actions that feel better and which are healthy:

- Call a positive friend on the phone
- Take a hot bath
- Read a book
- Listen to uplifting music
- Take a walk
- Engage in a hobby

Some people find it relaxing to paint small figures related to fantasy stories of dragons and knights. Others find listening to music enjoyable.

What small things might lift *your* mood?

2. Ignite small disciplines

I have a practice called: *"Do it just for the discipline."*

For example, on some days, when I return on a train after teaching college students during the day, I invite my sweetheart to take a walk. Sometimes she mentions that she did not sleep well or she has some other physical ailment. I ask, "How about a 10 minute walk? 5 minutes out and 5 minutes back just for the discipline of it."

The idea is to keep a good habit in place. When you condition yourself to automatically do a good habit, it becomes easier to get the task done.

3. Go for the spoonful not the bucket

Consider the power of *"Control Your Portions."*

At mealtimes, I use a small bowl. I can later choose to have a second helping or to avoid having a second helping.

Realize that *"more is not necessarily better."*

For example, eight days ago, I ate a Twinkie®—that is I ate one section of the two that come in a package. I had not had a Twinkie in over 15 years, but I remembered that the first two bites were great! However, I remembered that eating both sections made me feel uncomfortable because I knew it would negatively impact my health goals. This is related to my phrase: "It's just candy." By this I mean: there is nothing in the food selection that is good for my body.

Here's another example: about once every four months, I go to a supermarket and purchase two small legs of fried chicken. I do not buy a whole chicken. All the oil and breading that are part of fried chicken are not good for my body so I go for the small portion. Additionally, I make my eating of fried chicken an infrequent activity.

Recently, my sweetheart bought burritos for dinner. I admit it: A burrito is my kryptonite. Why? I usually eat the whole thing! Otherwise, my dinner portion is much smaller. Why? I want to keep my stomach smaller. Researchers mention that keeping a small stomach helps you feel full sooner.

4. Honor "Better than Zero"

The idea is that any activity is better than no activity. For example, I keep an Exercise log. Today so far, I've walked fast at Level 3 on my treadmill for 15 minutes. I've walked with my sweetheart for 30 minutes and I've done back and neck exercises. The day is not over yet, but this is a good start.

Consider doing this: Put this book down and go for an 8 minute walk. That small action will be *Better Than Zero.*

I use the phrase Better Than Zero to remind myself that "Any positive effort is progress. It all counts."

5. Take action with what you have

One year I had an injury to my ankle so I did the "bicycle

in the air" exercise. And I used a chair like a scooter.

My point is: Find a way to move and elevate your heart rate in some manner even if you are injured and temporarily cannot perform your preferred activity.

6. Employ the "Power of Declaring"

"When we get home, I'm getting on the treadmill for 10 minutes," I said to my sweetheart as we drove home from a restaurant. Upon arrival, I immediately entered our home and dashed upstairs and onto my treadmill.

I call this process "the Power of Declaring." In essence, I declared my intention. As a bonus: I had to live up to my declaration that I had voiced to my sweetheart.

How can you use the Power of Declaring in your daily life?

7. Note and regulate your Comfort Food

I'm not suggesting that you completely cut out your Comfort Food. It's not realistic, and besides, you could create resentment and an overpowering craving.

My comfort food is . . . wait for it . . . Ramen. I'm part Asian. I do not keep Ramen in the house. I have to make a choice and go buy One Package. Why? It's not real food. To me, it's "candy."

My concern is that if we completely cut out a comfort food selection it becomes an issue.

The concern about something becoming "too big an issue" reminds me of lunchtime on the set of a feature film I was directing. Actors and crew were gathered while we were eating. The topic of "have no TV set in the house" came up. Many of us thought that was a good idea. "Then the kids would have to do something active," one actress said.

Soon the lead actor voiced a different opinion: "In my

neighborhood, one house had no TV set. The two kids had a problem by not having a TV set in the house. Every time the kids went over to another child's house, did they play? No. They went straight to the television set because having no TV in the house was too big an issue. I didn't think much about the TV because it was just there in my home. But for these kids, having no TV became a problem. They couldn't keep up with the other kids because they never saw the shows other children at school were talking about."

So I'm using the above story as an analogy. If you completely cut out your comfort food, you're likely to make it into a big deal. You might even obsess over it.

On the other hand, you can take a moderate approach. For example, three days ago, I bought one package of Ramen. I know it's in the cupboard, but I haven't cooked it yet. It is no big deal. And the good news is: I do NOT have a habit of eating Ramen everyday.

Now it's your turn.

What are your comfort foods?

Can you keep them, for the most part, out of your home or at least hidden in a cupboard?

8. Use a pedometer

I wear a pedometer all day. This keeps fitness in my mind and it's certainly encouraging to see that I've walked 7,923 steps so far today.

It's reported that 10,000 steps a day are valuable for dropping weight. Many of us need to work up to the level of 10,000 steps.

One of my clients noted that he could leisurely walk 1,700 steps in 15 minutes or about 3,000 in 15 minutes at level 3 on his treadmill. We're looking at 9000 steps in 45 minutes at a relatively fast rate.

So walking 10,000 steps will take some time. The good news is that walking is easier on one's knees than running.

9. Place the "Worst First" task

I eat salad for breakfast. Why? Researchers note that willpower is like a muscle that is fresh early in the day, yet becomes "fatigued" by the end of the day.

In a way, eating salad has been a "worst first" task for me. The good news is that I do eat salad and support my great health. Even better, I reach for salad "by reflex" in the morning. Good habits are easier to maintain when you do NOT make the same decision again. Instead, you take positive action automatically.

Now it's your turn.

Is exercising your Worst First Task?

Is eating salad something that bothers you? Would you do better by eating salad earlier in the day?

* * * * * *

We will next look at two powerful topics related to dropping weight.

Drop Weight Using *Triple-Power Goals*

During a particularly stressful time when my elderly mother was in the hospital, I allowed myself to gain significant weight. My mother's hands and legs were not working, and it looked like she was near death. (Fortunately, a neurosurgeon's work restored my mother's health.)

At the time of my weight gain, I sat in the restroom and on rising I felt significant pain in my belly. This pain became an incentive to drop weight and get healthier. This pain relates to something I call a *Dark Boot Goal*. Imagine a big, dark boot kicking you in the rear and pushing you forward. The center of this situation is . . . Pain!

My point relates to something I observe as an executive coach: Many clients really get into action when pain pushes them.

Because of years of coaching clients, I developed what I call *Triple-Power Goals*:

- Golden Pull Goal
- Dark Boot Goal
- Green Tranquility Goal

We've discussed a *Dark Boot Goal*. You might have some significant pain that gives you real incentive to exercise more and modify your diet.

To empower yourself even more, pick a *Golden Pull Goal*. For some of us, we want better health so we can play with our children (or even grandchildren). The anticipation of joy and fun can be your Golden Pull Goal—it's positive and it pulls you to a great, enjoyable future.

After completing many projects whether it's a feature film or book, I've learned that achievements are *not* enough for a fulfilling life. So I include *Green Tranquility Goals*. Another way to express this type of goal is: a "Being Goal."

With a Being Goal, you enjoy inner peace and happiness by just being alive in the present moment.

For some people, a Being Goal is to simply enjoy a relaxed stroll in a park or somewhere in nature. Others feel a simple joy, relaxing in a hot bath. The idea is that you're enjoying the moment without making a big effort.

Now it's your turn.

Identify three forms of goals that relate to your drop-weight efforts.

What is a Dark Boot Goal related to your fitness efforts?

What is a Golden Pull Goal connected to your health-enhancing activities?

What is a Green Tranquility Goal so you enjoy feeling good in the moment?

A Look At the Spiritual Journey of Dropping Weight

"I hate my body!" my friend Adriana said about her body. It had ballooned outwards by 80 pounds.

As I reflected on her situation, I thought about the experience of hate versus love.

A number of authors suggest that hate arises from fear. Further, a number of learned people emphasize that, in regards to our spirituality, we have a choice in each given moment between love and fear.

Do we approach dropping weight because of hating our body or do we approach dropping weight because *we love ourselves and want to treat ourselves like a dear friend?*

This has a lot of consequences.

The truth is: Each of us is a constant work-in-progress. We do NOT really arrive on some permanent plateau. Depending on how you direct your focus, you could, at this moment, hate what your life has become. On the other hand, you could have a healthy and spiritual moment of being grateful for whatever good you have now. You have a choice to focus on the good from moment to moment. A helpful spiritual approach would be to live in gratitude *and* go for better.

We can take the view that this is an "AND-universe." So for the person who says, "I hate my body," what is the solution to hate? Gratitude.

What is the solution to fear? Gratitude *and* facing what ails us.

For example, I found myself wanting to make a big change in my diet. I came across some sources that suggest that artificial sweeteners can be worse than sugar because the body is "fooled" by them and the body can be harmed. It's reported that many obese people drink diet soda but the artificial sweeteners contribute to the calamity of gaining weight.

So I wanted to drop diet cola (full of caffeine and artificial sweeteners) from my diet. Yes, I wanted to drop weight.

Faced with trying to change my behavior, I could be harsh with myself. Or I could take a kind, spiritual approach.

So I looked for a gentle way for me to replace diet cola from my life. I found that I could buy simple carbonated water and add a bit of flavoring to it.

I was kind to myself and still gave myself the enjoyment of carbonated water.

Taking a kind, compassionate, spiritual approach to your drop-weight journey simply empowers you.

The idea of drop weight is: "I do not need that extra weight anymore. I can gently drop it from my life. I do not need to comfort myself with excess food or detrimental liquids."

Now it's your turn.

How can you be kind to yourself during your journey of dropping weight?

Principle:
Be kind to yourself and enhance your energy for your Drop-Weight Plan.

Power Question:
Are you putting energy into "I hate my body"? Can you shift to "I love myself and I am kind to myself on this health-enhancing journey"?

Highlights About San Francisco "I Lost My Thighs in San Francisco"

I grew up a chubby kid in San Francisco. One of the many things I enjoy about San Francisco is there are several scenic places to walk. *I know I became trim and stronger by walking a lot in San Francisco.* There are a lot of hills.

Walking Across the Golden Gate Bridge
My friends and I enjoy the amazing view from the bridge. Be prepared for a cold wind. Some people wear a hood because the wind can give them a headache. Still, gazing at the City or looking at ships and boats entering and leaving the San Francisco Bay provides a good time.

Ocean Beach
As a young filmmaker, I would often film parts of my film *True Hero* at the beach.

I attended Saint Ignatius College Preparatory, and the crew and I would walk to the beach.

Recently, I discovered that the sand dunes had been altered. When two friends and I walked on the sidewalk near the beach, sand slammed us in the face. Within two minutes, we said, "That's enough!" and we escaped to our car.

Here are some ways to enjoy the beach. Walk near the water and then you won't be as bothered by flying sand. Also, you can walk near the Cliff House Restaurant and still see the surf. If you stop for a meal in the Cliff House Restaurant, you can enjoy the view while gazing out big windows.

Lombard Street – "The Crookedest Street in the World"
I've walked on this famous, crooked street that's on a 27-degree angle.

It has eight hairpin turns, and you can enjoy landscaped flowerbeds.

You might want to Google this street and find out about when the street may have less traffic flow.

In any case, this is a notable landmark.

North Beach
Walking around here is interesting with various shops and places to eat. I enjoy a great pizza restaurant called, of course, North Beach Pizza. One night I gathered with friends at this restaurant and saw the final game of the World Series. As we stepped outside, we saw fireworks and then Koit Tower (which is shaped like the nozzle of a fire hose) lit up in a bright orange glow—the color worn by the winning San Francisco Giants.

A side note: After a gathering with friends, I had the idea for my musical called "San Francisco Pizza."

Mission District and Noe Valley
I grew up in the Mission District. And I was a nine-year-

old filmmaker who tossed lighter fluid and rubbing alcohol on the ground so I could do a scene with flames on the sidewalk. In the film, my character appears to pole-vault while his skateboard goes through the flames. [No one do a stunt like this!] This was my first brush with what I call "Film making fever." People will do dangerous things to get a shot. I have learned to be careful about that. In fact, I had the chance to hang from the side of a cliff for a shot in a feature film. It's amazing how a crew will follow the director. "Sure, he must know what he's doing." But instead, as the director, I simulated the shot with camera angles. (This was before computer generated visual effects.)

I would frequently walk up the 24th Street hill to Noe Valley to attend grammar school.

24th Street in Noe Valley has a sprinkling of small shops to view.

Golden Gate Park

As a young filmmaker, I loved filming in the park. If you are going to go off the path, be sure to bring some form of bug repellant. After a day of filming, I found myself covered in bug bites. Ugh.

Still, you can enjoy the paths and sidewalks, and Golden Gate Park does serve as an "oasis" in the middle of the City.

On Sundays, the park closes John F. Kennedy Drive to cars. John F. Kennedy Drive extends from Stanyan Street to the 20th Avenue area. Bicyclists and people out for a stroll, run or dash-on-rollerblades all take advantage of this special opportunity to enjoy the park.

Japanese Tea Garden (Golden Gate Park) and Japantown

The Tea Garden is small with many pretty details

including an amazingly steep bridge. Some distance away from the Golden Gate Park resides Japantown, which is small, too. The little shops remind me of certain places I saw in Tokyo. There's a little area that looks like a small "street" of old-time Japan (it's like a movie set) between a couple of restaurants. So it's almost like stepping into an entirely different country, hence the name: Japantown.

The Three Chinatowns

For about eight years, I had a Chinese girlfriend and we and her family were in a restaurant nearly every week.

Everyone knows about the **official Chinatown.** You'll see the Dragon Gate at its entrance. It is reported that The Republic of China (which resides in Taiwan) gifted the gate to the city of San Francisco in 1969.

The gate resembles similar ceremonial gates in Chinese villages. The ornate dragons and concrete guard dogs have a function, according to tradition, to keep evil spirits away.

The lampposts in this area look like pagodas with dragons' tails. A number of buildings have the distinctive Chinese style of architecture.

Tightly packed and colorful shops fill Chinatown, and lots of people buy produce, meat, and fish in the stores. It's a busy place!

Other Chinatown #1: It is the area around Green Apple Books (This is one of my favorite bookstores. I visit it anytime I'm in the area) at Clement and 6th Avenue. A number of shops and restaurants line the street. The Tat Wong Kung Fu School is located in this area.

Other Chinatown #2: It is the area around Irving and 19th Ave. When I think of Irving Street, I also recall the Shangrila Vegetarian Restaurant. This a Chinese eatery that serves noodle dishes and faux meats. They also serve other vegetarian, vegan and kosher meals.

The above details are just a sampling of varied places to walk in San Francisco. During my college years at Santa Clara University, I missed the diversity that I had experienced in San Francisco. Also the hills! Much of Silicon Valley is so flat! (My sweetheart just said, "That's why they call it a valley.")

I invite you to consider walking in your hometown "with the eyes of a tourist." By this I mean, take a moment and appreciate what you're seeing.

"We shall not cease from exploration, and the end of all our exploring will be to arrive where we started and know the place for the first time." - T. S. Eliot

BOOK TWO:
Energize through Happy Moments
(Happy Moments Empower You To Persist
with Your Drop-Weight Plan)

On a walking tour in San Francisco's Pacific Heights, I held my sweetheart's hand. She smiled at me as the Tour Guide said, "That's Chris Columbus' home." She knew that I had appreciated how Chris Columbus had directed *Mrs. Doubtfire,* starring Robin Williams and had written *Gremlins.*

Chris Columbus is, perhaps, best known for directing the first two *Harry Potter* feature films. He said, "I think there is a place for movies to leave people with a sense of hope."

I agree with him.

And I'll add that there is a place for getting exercise and having happy moments at the same time. A San Francisco Walking Tour provides such an opportunity.

* * *

"So on a scale of 1 to 10, how ready are you to do what it

takes to drop the extra weight?" I asked Serena, a client.

"4," she replied.

"4. Why is it not a 2?"

"What?" Serena asked.

"Why are you more ready than a 2? You said, '4.'" I confirmed.

"Because I don't want to be huge, and I don't want to get diabetes. My dad has diabetes. But I know what hard effort it's going to take . . ." she said.

Later, I reflected on this conversation, and I realized that *without some form of happiness in other areas of our lives*, we are likely to *fail in having the energy to persist* with our exercise/diet regimen.

So this book is going to step into a fresh area of discussion: *Experience Happiness WHILE You Drop Weight.*

This is a critical area for all of us who wish to do health-enhancing activities.

One of my friends, Max, told me, "I had a bad workout. My day is ruined."

"Ruined? The whole day?"

"Yeah! That's the only thing that is important to me."

On hearing this I realized that Max's focus for his life appeared *too small*. In fact, in a later conversation, I mentioned, "Perhaps, you might want to find someone new to serve?" I suggested this idea because I had the impression that over the years Max had lost his joy of living. Later, he confirmed this impression when he said, "Where did it go? In the 80's I used to be enthusiastic about things."

This is a prime area of concern. You need personal energy and some joy in your life so that you have the strength to persist through pain (whether it's some hunger pangs or the difficulties that arise with continued exercise).

As one of my editors points out: Emotional pain can drive

one to eat excessively.

So how do you deal with emotional pain? For many of us, having a refuge in trusted friends, family or even a therapist can be crucial.

Still, it's vital to observe that having some happy moments each day is critical to enhancing our reservoir of personal energy and willpower.

Any journey of dropping weight is going to have times where things slow down and our progress seems to have ended. Frustration can knock us out of the process IF we do not have sources of happiness elsewhere in our lives.

That's an essential part of the reason I'm including this section on Happiness in this book.

Your diet and exercise do NOT exist separately from the rest of your life. **In fact the rest of your life, when nurtured, can support your weight-dropping goals.**

Happiness can be a wonderful support and source of energy so you persist and continue to make progress with your weight dropping journey even when the road is fraught with potholes and bumps.

How to Have Your Brain Increase Your Happiness

"I don't sing because I'm happy; I'm happy because I sing."
— William James

The above quote is a classic one that reminds us: Our actions can guide us to feeling better. At the same time, our thoughts can support us to feel better.

Certain thoughts arise automatically and if we remain in the pattern of *draining-thoughts,* we can fall into a low mood. Such a low mood can drain our energy and we may fall into two behaviors: a) not moving/not exercising or b) eating comfort food.

What thought can knock you down into a low mood? A thought tinged with perfectionism.

About Perfectionism:

Perfectionism can torpedo your Drop-Weight Plan and actions. I'll say it here: I do not have a "perfect body." Sometimes I glance at my belly and go, "Looks good for a guy in his 50's." My belly is significantly trimmer than a number of 50 year-olds I see, but sometimes, if I eat some pizza, I don't like what it does to my belly area.

Focus on my belly is a focus of perfectionist-thoughts for me. But *I've learned to shift* my focus to *what I can do*. I still do martial arts kicks, sit-ups, pushups, and I lift weights. Just not as much as a professional athlete. I can still do the moves in a movie fight scene if I would start to make a new film. (I've been a lead actor in two feature films who has done martial art fight scenes.)

I share my two forms of thoughts (perfectionism and "what I can do") to demonstrate that I face the problems that perfectionism brings, too.

My point in sharing this is: Identify your draining-thoughts and your perfectionism-thoughts. And then shift to *Empowering Thoughts*. **This is the way to have your brain increase your happiness, and in turn, increase your personal energy.** Identify what you can do, what progress you're making and *what you are able to do*. For example, one of my friends, Matilda, found that she was huffing and puffing after merely walking up stairs. It was clear that she wanted to drop weight so that merely walking up stairs would not be a tough part of her day.

Matilda started easy. In fact, I have an idea I call "The Easy Part Start." She started by walking around her block. Then she added walking up a medium hill. Within months, she was hiking in the hills near her home.

Now we will explore 12 Topics which will help you continue with your Drop-Weight Plan WHILE you support your personal happiness.

More moments of happiness lead to more personal energy that you can apply to your Drop-Weight Plan.

Book Two / Topic #1

I'm sharing this next article because dropping weight includes setting a goal or a series goals. Many of us hate setting goals because we've failed in the past. Such pain can lead us to simply avoid setting a new, empowering goal.

But this is NOT for you.

Improve your life; the first step is to study how to set *better* goals.

How You Can Overcome Fear and Achieve Goals that Make a Big Difference

"No! I hate goals," my friend Serena told me. She had endured years of yo-yo dieting. Her weight plummeting and rising up to a worse level than before the diet.

Have you been afraid of setting an ambitious goal and then failing—and then facing humiliation?

Success and fulfillment arise, in part, due to a strategic approach to goal setting and goal-achievement. We'll use the A.I.M. process:

A – adjust for the long game
I – intensify systems
M – measure the empowering way

1. Adjust for the long game

Some people avoid goal-setting because they want to avoid pain in the forms of disappointment, frustration and embarrassment.

The truth is everyone faces some frustration and disappointment even if they are just trying to have a quiet life. But the important point is that without goal setting and goal-achievement, you will miss out on feeling good about yourself and about your life in general. Setting a personal goal and making progress yields your feeling hopeful!

Look at "the long game." By this I mean, look at building your whole life, not just some temporary setbacks that you might call failures.

For example, among my 27 books on Amazon.com, three of them do not sell at all. Some might call those books failures. Instead, I look upon those books (and writing them) as stepping stones. To this day, I use my research and writing from those books every semester when I teach graduate students and college students. So nothing was lost.

Writing those books was part of my "long game" plan. In writing 27 books, I've done a lot of research, thinking and creating of material. I bring these developments to every speech I give.

Now it's your turn.

How can you set a small goal and remind yourself that it's all part of your life-path? Remember small steps add up for your better life.

2. Intensify systems

Instead of setting a tough goal, gritting your teeth and hoping to stay on your vigorous schedule, place a new system into your life. That is, create a system for taking action that becomes a natural part of your day.

For example: recently, a colleague asked me to help her make sure that she rehearses enough for her next presentation.

I asked, "What do you do everyday?"

"Brush my teeth," she replied.

"How about rehearsing your speech for three minutes immediately after you complete brushing your teeth?" I suggested.

"I could do that," she replied.

Then I suggested that she set up a reward for herself when she completes three sessions of rehearsal.

Now, she gained an empowering system possessing both specific actions and rewards.

Now it's your turn.

What do you want to make sure that you do on a daily basis? How can you reward yourself for taking action?

3. Measure the empowering way

Some people find it too painful to endure the emotional roller-coaster of weighing themselves everyday. A solution is to check one's weight only once a week.

Still, we do well when we focus on three important details about measuring: a) what, b) when, and c) meaning

For example, when I wanted to drop weight, I had these details:

1) *What?* What is my belt measurement? (I was glad when I had slimmed down to three notches slimmer on the belt.)

2) *When?* I programmed weighing myself once a week.

3) *Meaning:* The belt measurement was more important to me than the weight number because I was also doing weight training. Weight training builds muscle, and muscle fibers weigh more than fat or other tissues. So, for me, the weight number was NOT the only meaningful measurement.

Now it's your turn.

How can you identify the three elements (what, when, and meaning) of using empowering measurement? What will you measure? How often? And what does the measurement really mean towards your accomplishing your larger goal?

A Word about Setting a Goal and Feeling Embarrassed

My friend "Jackson" set a goal of dropping 20 pounds in 90 days. His result? Only 5 pounds. He was truly disappointed.

To be supportive, I mentioned the concept of a "growth mindset" (a concept developed by author/researcher Carol S. Dweck.)

When we have a growth mindset, we take a "failure" or setback as a natural part of the process. My friend only dropped 5 pounds. That's in the right direction! Now, he can look over his measurements. Did he walk 10,000 steps each day? No. Perhaps, that's a big part of how he did not achieve his 20 pound weight loss goal.

As a result, he can start again and change his behaviors. He can improve his approach and get better and better results. He can use a growth mindset.

When you set goals, sometimes, you will be disappointed. Sometimes, you may even appear to fail—in front of others. In my video "How to Believe in Yourself When Others Don't" [at YouTube.com type in "Tom Marcoux great year" to view the 7 min video—or visit OptiRealist.com], I said, "Measure by your heart, not by their approval." It's understandable to feel embarrassed when you seem to fall short of a goal. There are a number of ways to deal with this. *One:* Only tell supportive people about your goal. *Two:* Hold strong and realize that no matter what you do or do not do, someone will criticize you. It's just a fact of life. Eleanor Roosevelt said: "Do what you feel in your heart to be right— for you'll be criticized anyway." So take the calculated risk. Create some forward motion in your life. Truly, you are the only one who really cares about what good you can create in your own life.

When I talk about overcoming fear, I mean that you do not let fear stop you from taking action. So choose your goal. Choose carefully with whom you share your goal. And even when others criticize, be your own cheerleader because you have the courage to step forward, learn and keep going.

I invite you to make your own standards (what is in your heart) more important than what others say. Tell yourself (and even sometimes tell others), "I'm making progress. I'm learning as I go. I'm getting better at this. I have a good trend going."

Consider setting goals according to the A.I.M. process:

A – adjust for the long game
I – intensify systems
M – measure the empowering way

Each day you can make progress.
I say that any step forward is *Better Than Zero*.
The best to you on your journey.

We learned strategies for setting better goals and taking action in the above article.

Principle:
Set goals that serve you long term on your life-path.

Power Question:

Will you set goals and keep up your morale by telling yourself "I'm making progress; I'm getting better at this; I have a good trend going"?

Book Two / Topic #2

We now turn to the below article because our discussion in this section is about happiness. I've learned that happiness is not a mere fleeting feeling of pleasure. It's more about being aligned with what is good inside you. My clients report that they experience more moments of authentic happiness when they are supportive to other people. In essence, when you experience authentic happiness, you have more personal energy to devote to staying on course with your Drop-Weight Plan.

How to Be Awake and Alive in this Present Moment

The film brought tears to my eyes. Why? Here were characters trying to do something good—something that could raise human beings to a higher level of living, to more kindness, courage, loyalty and love.

Isn't that worth crying about and doing something about?

As a writer of books and as a speaker, I get a number of opportunities to express the truth as I've learned it so far. Here's a truth that I know: *One of the kindest things each of us can do is listen, truly listen to another person.*

But there are things in our way. Fear is a big one. We're so preoccupied with trying to survive that we're running fast, doing what we think will help us survive. But here's another truth that I know. **Surviving is NOT enough. We're here to live.**

I often write about the value of our nurturing ourselves. Why? So we can be stronger. The reason? So we can really be awake and alive in this present moment.

Years ago, I renamed one of my first books to the title of *Be Heard and Be Trusted* (3rd Edition, 15th Anniversary). That's the name of my blog, too. I was so excited when that title arose in my thoughts.

Let's face it: Each of us wants to be heard. And that's the gift you can give. Assure another person that *you are really listening to his or her feelings and concerns. You listen closely to learn what is really in the person's heart.*

By the way, here are a few tips to help you listen better. Observe yourself. Are you letting the reflex to judge someone's words to block your listening?

Recently, I did one of the toughest things in my life.

My father, now in his 70s, in recent years has been simply cruel to family members—saying mean words and then simply ignoring family members.

Six days ago, my father actually called me over to talk with him, just as I was finishing a visit with my mother who was recovering from surgery. My father jabbed at me with his words. He reiterated his usual complaints and even disparaging remarks about family members. But there were just a few seconds of a quieter tone.

Even so, it took so much energy for me to stand there and listen to him. I did not jump in and refute his comments. I heard him out. I forced myself to look in his eyes while he spoke.

He saw that I was paying attention.

I did my best to listen.

I gave my father the gift of my listening.

A gift he has not given, and maybe cannot give, to me and others.

Still, I listened.

* * * *

When we listen to someone, we can do a great kindness: Provide a *Reflective Reply*. That is, respond to the person in a way that assures them that you heard their feelings.

You can say something like:

- That sounds frustrating.
- That sounds disappointing.
- That sounds intense. How did you feel about it?

Sometimes, you might follow-up with: "Is there some way I can help with that?"

Yes—there are big things to be done.

I always remember this quote:

"Never doubt that a small group of thoughtful, committed citizens can change the world; indeed, it's the only thing that ever has." – Margaret Mead

And here's something I also never doubt.

To make things better, we need to push aside distractions of the ego and really listen to the person right in front of us.

That may not get you a Nobel Prize.

But it just might give you the feeling of warmth in your heart and a good night's sleep.

"You must be the change you wish to see in the world."
– Mahatma Gandhi

Practice being compassionate toward yourself and spread such compassion to the person next to you.

By the way, keep listening to your own heart.

"Don't ask what the world needs. Ask what makes you come alive, and go do it. Because what the world needs is people who have come alive." – Howard Thurman

We learned about the gift of listening and *really living* in the above article.

Principle:
Give the gift of listening and feel truly alive.

Power Question:
Will you practice the process of providing a *Reflective Reply?*

We now turn to this next article by Patricia Fripp because eye contact is a vital element of communication. Researchers note that numerous people report that 80% of their happiness is related to their relationships. Such relationships are enhanced by listening and eye contact (as I mentioned my giving my father eye contact in my above article). Listening and eye contact are vital parts of making other people feel important. I emphasize with clients and college students: *When you're listening, you're winning.*

5 Tips for How to Connect with Eye Contact
by Patricia Fripp, CSP, CPAE

Generally speaking, the longer the eye contact between two people, the greater the intimacy is developed. In a business, sales and speech situation, look at members of your audience for a thought, phrase or idea. If you are sitting at a boardroom table, make sure you share eye contact with everyone.

Others rarely interrupt two people engaged in a conversation if they have consistent eye contact. Through observing eye contact, others, well at least thoughtful ones, can tell if it is okay to join in the conversation.

Pupils enlarge when people are talking about things that bring them joy or happiness. They often contract when discussing issues that bring them sadness. In a conversation at a networking or social event, I always like to ask questions of interest to my conversation partner. It helps add to their, "I enjoyed meeting that person," feeling.

The longer your eye contact, the more self-esteem you are perceived to have.

The more eye contact you can maintain, the higher self-esteem you are perceived to have.

Being perceived as more likable gives you an unfair advantage in business. And we all want an unfair advantage to success! Eye contact is an important way to build this emotional bond and likeability.

* * *

Being perceived as a dynamic, inspiring, and persuasive communicator is a matter of business life and death! Get 24/7 access to executive speech coach and sales presentation skills expert Patricia Fripp when you sign up for FrippVT today at www.FrippVT.com.

Patricia Fripp, CSP, CPAE is an award-winning keynote speaker, business presentation expert, sales presentation skills trainer, and in-demand speech coach to executives and celebrity speakers and known as "the speaker's speaker." *Meetings & Conventions* magazine named her "One of the 10 most electrifying speakers in North America." Fortune 500 companies maximize their investment by engaging Patricia for the keynote, breakout sessions, and to coach their executives on their presentations. Patricia is known for simplifying and demystifying the process of designing and delivering powerful keynote speeches and sales presentations.

www.frippvt.com, prfripp@fripp.com, (415) 753-6556
Patricia Fripp, "Improving business one presentation at a time."

Book Two / Topic #3

I'm sharing the next article because it provides vital insights about *developing a system of behavior change.* Dropping weight requires that we use a system *we customize.* The system only works when it deeply connects with the individual.

How to Make the Best Day of Your Life

"I'm feeling so good. I didn't think I could do this. But today, I'm starring in my own film. Thanks, Tom, for believing in me," James said, from his chair on the set of a short film.

The first time I encouraged James was when he attended a class I held. We remained in contact and I further encouraged him to take steps forward.

When I give a keynote address, sometimes the meeting planner uses the words "motivational speaker." I'm okay with those words, but I prefer "**Transformational Speaker** or **Transformational Coach.**"

How do I help people make a Big Difference in their life? It comes down to actual systems of behavior change.

To have the *Best Day of your life* often requires that you create new habits and that you prepare yourself. Before a big day, one has to put things into place. For example, James had to create a new habit of writing his script for his film—before he could get onto the set and film it.

Imagine what would be *The Best Day of Your Life.* Would you be doing something fulfilling as your job?—acting, singing, writing? Would you be on an amazing vacation with someone you love?

To help clients and audiences raise their level of success and happiness, I innovated something I call *"The Celebrate Habits Method."*

In part, it's based on three elements of the C.A.N. process:

C – concentrate when you're strong
A – arrange connections
N – nurture new results

When you use the three elements of C.A.N., you're able to create lasting, positive habits. Such habits lead to *transforming your life*—not just small improvements.

1. Concentrate when you're strong

Research noted at Stanford University emphasizes that willpower acts like a muscle. Many people find that their willpower is stronger earlier in the day. For example, my clients and I use the practice of *"Worst First"*—that is, we do the toughest task earlier in the day when we're fresh. Some people get a "second wind" in the afternoon, so that may be the best time for them to schedule their toughest task.

When are you fresh and strong? Can you schedule your new task (for your new habit) then?

By the way, performing tough tasks when you are fresh and strong allows you to complete the task faster and with greater ease. You *Celebrate your victory* and feel great!

2. Arrange connections

To ensure that you do your new behavior, connect it to something that you already do naturally. This is *connecting the task to your "natural flow of the day."* For example, in the car, when returning from a restaurant, I announce to my sweetie, "I'm getting on the treadmill immediately when we get home."

The strategy here is: I'm already in motion as I enter the house so I simply go straight to the treadmill.

What can you connect to your new behavior? Do you surf the Internet everyday? How about using a stationary bicycle while you surf the 'Net?

3. Nurture new results

To set positive habits in place and get new, better results, you simply need more energy. Become strategic in how you enhance and support your personal energy. Some of my clients log their sleep. If they miss getting rest, they will take extra care to get more sleep on a subsequent day.

Another way to nurture new results is to *measure your progress.*

For example, I measure my progress with a log book that I keep next to my computer monitor. The log book also serves as a *positive trigger.* In this way, I do back exercises everyday because the log book triggers me to do the exercise. I measure how many sit-ups, pushups, martial arts moves and weight-training sessions I accomplish each week. My phrase is: *Keep score and achieve more.*

I also suggest: **You can expect what you inspect.** Again, measuring efforts and results helps you ultimately transform your life.

How can you nurture yourself and enhance your personal energy?

How can you measure your daily efforts and subsequent results?

I designate the C.A.N. process as part of my *Celebrate Habits Method* because **installing positive habits can bring you to a higher level of success and happiness**—beyond your first imaginings.

Get started today.

We learned how to consistently change our behaviors in the above article. Working with this inspiration, I'll now provide you with a *principle* and *power question.*

Principle:
Keep score and achieve more.

Power Question:
How will you measure or log your daily progress?

Book Two / Topic #4

We now turn to this article because many of us miss out on happiness due to being pushed and pulled by other people and outside forces. To do better, we'll focus on tools to help you rise to higher levels of happiness and success.

Use the Secret Success Equation and Rise When the World Holds You Back

Do you have a plan for rising after the world slams you down? Every successful person I've interviewed has demonstrated the independence of thought and habit to rise up even when others are actively disrupting their positive efforts. I've developed a **"Secret Equation of Happiness and Success"** to vividly demonstrate the Truth of what's going on and how you can protect yourself and triumph!

The World's Weapons Against Your Ability to Truly Enjoy Life:
- Distraction is -2
- Indifference is -2
- Contempt is -2

Your Tools to Take Your Life to Higher Levels of Success and Happiness

- Focus is +3
- Your Heartfelt Interest is +3
- Your Own Approval is +3

So it's 9 − 6 = 3

That's the *Plus-3 Edge for Happiness and Success*

Do NOT let the world beat you down and steal your dream.

Let's explore this further.

1. Focus
(overcome distraction)

"You want to watch this TV show?" called one of my family members. And it was the easiest thing in the world for me to sit down and watch another television program. But I reminded myself: "Focus. Make some progress."

I am all for a balance of leisure and activity. However, I am really conscious of how some people I know simply do not have powerful goals and dreams. These individuals simply drift, trying to stay comfortable.

But it's worse than that: Certain people exhibit the infamous "crab mentality." One way to describe this is: "If I can't have it, neither can you." In a pot of boiling water, crabs hold each other down and they all die! If they simply did not interfere with each other, they'd all escape and live.

Be conscious of how some friends and even some family members will distract you: more food when you're on a diet . . . or . . . TV when you want to write your novel.

Who in your life is distracting you and pulling you away from your highest good? Is it time to spend less time with that person?

2. Your Heartfelt Interest
(overcome indifference)

Over the years, my father has shut down conversations. If I'm excited about progress on my graphic novel series, *Jack AngelSword*, he has simply said, "Yeah. You could do that many ways." And then he shifts into complaining about something. He allows no space for me to express my thoughts or feelings.

His indifference causes pain for family members. As a result, I've learned to go my own way and support my own Heartfelt Interest.

Have you wasted your time or effort trying to get a loved one to listen to what you're interested in? Do you need to find "a new tribe" — people who share your real interests?

Your Own Approval
(overcome contempt)

My client Sarah showed her sister Tanya some first drawings for her own planned fantasy series of books.

"They're not very good, are they?" Tanya emphasized.

Sarah later said, "Tanya just shut me down. Not even a 'hey, you're making progress on that.'"

Sarah needs to celebrate her progress and to stop waiting for Tanya's approval.

This reminds me of the cherished words from author Marianne Williamson: *"Your playing small does not serve the world. There is nothing enlightened about shrinking so that other people won't feel insecure around you. We were born to make manifest the glory of God within us."*

Put more energy into expressing yourself and feeling good about such expression. Instead of worrying about how other people will react to your work, be sure to enjoy your own process.

"If you always do what interests you, at least one person is pleased." – Katharine Hepburn

You need to build yourself up and nurture yourself.

"You cannot help small [people] by tearing down big [people].
You cannot strengthen the weak by weakening the strong . . .
You cannot build character and courage by taking away

[people's] initiative and independence." – William Boetcker

It's interesting that the above quote is often misattributed to Abraham Lincoln. Lincoln is famous for enduring numerous failures and setbacks. He lost several elections and even endured a nervous breakdown. Still, *he acted on his own initiative* again and again. He came back to win the office of the U.S. presidency.

Build your own strength by focusing on what moves your heart—the source of your personal initiative.

Remember this equation:

Focus + Your Heartfelt Interest + Your Own Approval = Success and Happiness

The best to you.

We learned about outside forces that poison our happiness and how to combat them in the above article.

Principle:
When you develop your own standards and focus on your own approval, other people cannot control you with their contempt.

Power Questions:
What are you own standards? What means most to you? How can you separate that from seeking anyone else's approval?

Book Two / Topic #5

I am sharing this next article because when many of us are worried or in pain we may reach for food for comfort. There is an alternative. Learn to purposely shift your thoughts in an empowering direction. Happiness is *not* found in an absence of uncertainty or pain; life confronts us with uncertainty frequently. We're called to become skillful about uncertainty. As I've mentioned earlier, happiness is more than a fleeting feeling. It's really a healthy approach to life. Here's the process:

How You Can Deal Well with Uncertainty

My family member had not slept for more than 24 hours. She had promised me that she'd call another family member to retrieve her from the hospital. That was the plan. I slept with my cell phone near my head.

Upon awakening, I heard that she had driven herself home from the hospital.

When I saw her, I gave her a hug and said, "I'm glad you're safe."

Inside I felt an emotional tumble like an operating dryer.

I realized that I needed to fall back on methods to deal with uncertainty. Why uncertainty? Because she was likely to drive again in the future when she was too tired. Yes— she's stubborn.

Why does this bother me? Too many people I know (or have heard about) have died while driving while tired. For example, one of the production team members who worked on James Cameron's feature film *TITANIC* **died** while driving when too tired. He could have slept in his office, but no—he drove his car while he was too tired and he drifted off the road to his death.

By the way, being too tired can impair one's ability to make a good decision.

So life makes us face other people's stubborn behaviors and events that bring up worry and feelings of uncertainty.

My clients and I have come up with phrases that help us turn the direction of our worried-thoughts. Here are some examples:

- With God, I can handle this.
- I've endured tough times before. I'll endure, I'll learn. I'll get deeper.
- I am Spirit having a human experience.
- I'm focusing on *This Present Moment.*

The truth is: as human beings, we'll all get our share of problems and times for grieving. The solution is to stay in *This Present Moment* . . . instead of getting stuck and lost in worries of the future.

I've learned that much of the pain of uncertainty is about getting stuck in "catastrophe-thinking." (That's ruminating about potential catastrophes.)

The solution is to shift out of catastrophe-thinking.

I'm certainly concerned about my family member being safe and driving when fresh and wide awake. However, when it comes to the behavior of another human being, particularly an adult, we all have limited influence.

To shift out of catastrophe-thinking, I have used this thought: "I don't run that show."

This reminds me that my family member runs her own life.

Also, Higher Power runs the universe. **I don't run that show.**

Many of us turn to the phrase: *Let Go, Let God.*

To deal well with uncertainty, pick your next thought. Pick your focus.

Again, consider these phrases:

- Let Go, Let God.
- I don't run that show.
- With God, I can handle this.
- I've endured tough times before. I'll endure, I'll learn. I'll get deeper.
- I am Spirit having a human experience.
- I'm focusing on *This Present Moment.*

Living at the top of your game involves taking appropriate risks. To do that, you need to be able to think clearly. Pay attention to what helps you calm down.

Some of my clients, just before they go to sleep, ask a question:

Why is it easy for me to fall asleep?

Because I'm safe. Because God has a plan for me.

Because I'll feel refreshed on waking up tomorrow.

I'll wake up thinking: "Thank you, God for this new day for love, prosperity and excellent health."

We learned how to deal with uncertainty in the above article.

Principle:

Develop your skills to face uncertainty and make the most of the present moment.

Power Question:

What phrase will you use to help you shift your focus from disquieting thoughts? Will you try "Let go, Let God" or something like "I don't run that show"?

Book Two / Topic #6

I'm sharing this next article because you will truly enhance your happiness with two actions: a) support the work of the Law of Attraction in your life and b) overcome self-sabotage.

Law of Attraction and How You Can Overcome Self-Sabotage

Adriana knows that if she attends a networking event on Tuesday, she will increase her circle of contacts. But she engages in self-sabotage by staying awake too late on Monday night. She makes herself too tired on Tuesday to attend the networking event, and so she misses her opportunity to expand her networking circle of contacts. Why does she engage in self-sabotage?

That *is* the question: Why do we sabotage ourselves? Much of it arises from the conditioning that we endured as a younger person. As children we do not realize the harm created by limiting beliefs (foisted on us by parents and guardians). As we grow up, the beliefs are simply what we know.

The Law of Attraction is hampered by the mixed signals we send into the universe when we're restrained by limiting beliefs, confusion and fear of uncertainty.

(By the way, the Law of Attraction refers to the universal principle that you attract what you think about most.)

As I mentioned above, these are the particular, insidious elements:

1) Limiting beliefs
2) Confusion

3) Fear of uncertainty

1) Limiting beliefs

Just a few minutes ago, a friend was driving her car and said to me, "Oh, no! We're going to catch all the red lights." I replied, "I don't know that; we haven't arrived at each light yet."

A big problem with a limiting belief is that it *drains* your energy. The phrase "We're going to catch all the red lights" causes stress, and the phrase may be wrong!

A limiting belief can even cause you pain because a limiting belief can wind up your body with adrenaline.

One of my friends "Cindy" gets chest pains when she hears certain words. For example, she talked with her therapist and felt pain when asked, "Who are you pleasing too much?"

So Cindy holds two limiting beliefs: 1) If I take care of myself and take a few nights to relax, some people will not like me because I'm not helping them, and 2) my health is really fragile.

Both limiting beliefs box her in so she does *not* do certain activities.

In this way, limiting beliefs are a big part of her self-sabotaging actions and self-sabotaging inactivity.

The solution includes taking a good look at your beliefs. Talk about them. Ask yourself: Is this belief true for me now—as an adult? Was this belief just something I constructed when I was afraid as a child?

For example, author Lois P. Frankel wrote books called *Nice Girls Don't Get the Corner Office* and *Nice Girls Don't Get Rich.* Lois' point is that "being a nice girl" was something that was okay for childhood, but what's better now is "being a Strong Woman."

Now it's your turn.

In your journal, write down five of your beliefs. Now look at them carefully. Does each belief help you? Is the belief even true for you now? Could you hold a better belief?

Some people mindlessly parrot a comment "money is the root of all evil."

Instead of that, I say, "Money is a tool I use well for the benefit of all involved." I prefer my *Expansive Belief.*

2) Confusion

Confusion arises from mixed thoughts and mixed feelings. Here are examples:

- I want this, but I don't deserve it.
- I want this, but I'm afraid that things will get worse.

Sometimes, our confusion and mixed feelings lie below the surface in our subconscious mind. To get at such subconscious turmoil and to shine some light on the elements, we can talk about the details with someone we trust. We need a session in which we talk and the other person simply listens and does not offer comments. It could help if the friend or counselor writes down some notes. Then, the friend could read back something we say. This helps because sometimes we say something, but we do not really notice the kernel of truth in our words. Many of us just gloss over details, hopping from topic to topic. *The friend could get us to pause and reflect on something we said.*

Another way to get at our subconscious beliefs and feelings is through drawing or assembling images we find in magazines. Do the process quickly and see what you find on the paper.

I once responded to a direction in a workbook: "Draw a sketch of your parents." I drew a volcano to represent my father. And I drew an invisible woman (made of dashes instead of lines) to represent my mother. I learned much from those sketches.

Now it's your turn.

Pick a method: Sketch an image or assemble pictures from magazines to represent what your mind is thinking in the moment.

See what your images bring up in terms of your feelings and thoughts.

A solution: Imagine that this is an "AND universe."

Here are examples:

- *I feel "I want this, but I don't deserve it."* I can take steps forward AND I can make the project serve people. So I can get what I want AND by serving others, I will feel that the project is worthwhile.

- *I feel "I want this, but I'm afraid that things will get worse.* I can take small steps forward. I can get expert advice. I can get training so that I'm stronger in this area of work. AND I can look at what might go wrong. AND I can take steps so I can adapt to anything that may go wrong. AND I can learn from the journey.

Write down your own "AND-possibilities."

3) Fear of uncertainty

Do the thing you fear and the death of fear is certain.

– Ralph Waldo Emerson

I've done many things that inspired fear in me: first time directing a feature film, first time giving a speech to 697 people, and first time writing a book.

I might hesitate to say that my fear "died."

What did die was my being sabotaged by fear. Instead of being frozen by fear, I stepped forward.

That's an important realization.

Of my 27 books, about three do *not* sell. So I've endured "failure" with writing a book that does not find an audience.

I've learned to face the uncertainty and NOT let the uncertainty shut down my activity or creativity.

Now it's your turn.

Does feeling uncertain and feeling fear stop you in your tracks? Is there something you can make More Important than fear? Write your thoughts and feelings in your journal.

"Courage is not the absence of fear but rather the judgment that something is more important than fear." – Meg Cabot

The "This or Better" Solution

If you have a spiritual path, you could say this prayer that invokes the Law of Attraction.

"Please help me make _____ happen in my life. Thank you for supporting me on this path. I want ____ . . . I want this or better. Thank you."

The idea of the Law of Attraction is that you attract what you think about most.

A good plan is to get clear on what you want and still make space so the universe delivers what you want **or better.**

We learned about overcoming self-sabotage in the above article.

Principle:

Identify your limiting beliefs and work to focus on thoughts that empower you.

Power Questions:

What is one of your limiting beliefs? How can you turn

that around? Ask yourself: Is this belief true for me now—as an adult? Was this belief just something I constructed when I was afraid as a child?

Finally, ask yourself: "What belief would help me focus on positive opportunities?"

Book Two / Topic #7

We now turn to this next article because we often feel truly happy when we're in motion and taking positive steps to manifest what we want deep in our heart.

6. Law of Attraction and Your Essence of Power

"I've tried the Law of Attraction and 'Ask, Believe, Receive'—and I've received nothing!" Sam complained bitterly. "I hear you," I replied, "There is another detail: It's your Essence of Power."

"What's that?" Sam asked.

"It's what I call 'Devoted Action,'" I continued.

Sitting and meditating and "asking and believing (the traditional elements that people mention when talking about the Law of Attraction)" are only a part of the equation. There is another element that needs to be added: **Action is Crucial.** A *specific* form of action is needed. I call it *Devoted Action* because it is *focused* action for *what your heart really wants.*

"I want more money," Tabitha says. But she also says, "Rich people made their money hurting others." So what does she *really* want? Further in the discussion, she comes to the realization that she just wants the pain of having bills to stop. AND, she wants to think of herself as a good person. Unfortunately she has a Limiting Belief about wealth. In her childhood, she started, deep down, associating "more money" with "bad people."

To counter that debilitating thought, I have my own focus-point: **"Money is a tool I use well for the benefit of all involved."**

How do I use money well? Through Devoted Action. I pay close attention to budgets and value. Instead of the words Devoted Action, other people use the word "discipline."

"There are two types of pain you will go through in life, the pain of discipline and the pain of regret. Discipline weighs ounces while regret weighs tons." – Jim Rohn

So the question is "How is Devoted Action your Essence of Power?"

The answer relates to how the universe watches to see if you're serious about something. In some ways, the universe operates like the counter at a diner. You tell the waitperson your order. Simply. Forthrightly. Politely. That is, you **take action.**

If you do not tell your order, you do not get breakfast.

Similarly, **Devoted Action or "disciplined action" is your way of telling the universe: "Look I want THIS so much that I'm taking action for it!"**

There is *another element* to this process. We'll go back to the diner metaphor and expand upon it: It's like the cook saying, "You want eggs? Go get the carton of eggs in the refrigerator." Since you like how this cook prepares eggs, you do not hesitate. Off you go to get and return with the eggs.

So if you want the Law of Attraction to truly and quickly work for you, identify what disciplined action (or "Devoted Action"), you need to do. And do it.

Then you will start seeing excellent results.

(For more on the Law of Attraction plus the Law of Being and the Law of Creation, please see my book *Yes! Secrets for Your Best Life—Law of Attraction: Plus Hidden Power Increases Your Success and Happiness.*)

We learned about devoted action in the above article.

Principle:
Devoted Action takes you from asking and believing to actually manifesting what you want in life.

Power Question:
How can you move to Devoted Action and make efforts to manifest what you want?

Book Two / Topic #8

I'm now sharing this next article because it's easy for us to miss seeing how the seeds of our happiness are quietly blooming even during tough times. It all adds up to make you stronger and ultimately happier.

How You Can Make Your Bright Future— The Truth!

Want to hear what every successful person I've interviewed has told me? Their theme comes down to "I was afraid but I took steps forward that were immediately in front of me. Still, **it all added up.** Things I did in the present set up a brighter future—better than I imagined."

We'll focus on two vital questions:

- How can I take action today and build my personal brand?
- How can I stay aware of potential opportunities— even surprising ones?

These two questions became vivid in my mind as I thought about how I'm scheduled to give a keynote address in Oregon, USA, later this year. The leadership of the conference invited me to provide information about my speech: "The 3 C's of Success: Seize Your Advantage."

It became So Clear to me that I've been training my whole life to give this keynote address!

Here's information from the conference's website:
"Tom Marcoux speaks on *The 3 C's of Success:*

- Charisma
- Confidence

- Control of Time

Speaker-Author Tom Marcoux is uniquely qualified to guide YOU to higher levels of success and fulfillment.

- *Charisma* – Marcoux has served as a guest lecturer to MBA Students at STANFORD UNIVERSITY, guiding the students in making great first impressions (and improving time management skills). Author of a number of books on charisma including: *Create Your Best Life: Unleash Your Charisma and Confidence to Change the World* and *Be Heard and Be Trusted* (15th Anniversary, 3rd edition). Tom's new book is *Now You See Me – Make a Great First Impression and Use Secrets of Power Networking*.
- *Confidence* – CEO, a "Best of the Best" award-winning professional speaker and 14 year member of the National Speakers Association, and six-time speaker at the National Association of Broadcasters Conference, Las Vegas . . . Marcoux is a motion picture director, producer and actor.
- *Control of Time* – Marcoux is the author of 27 books sold in 15 countries including *Power Time Management: More Time, Less Stress and Zero Procrastination.*

'I started as a shy, nine-year-old boy, shaking as I played the piano for 31 seniors at a retirement home. I worked with coaches and mentors so that I could direct feature films and energize audiences of hundreds of people. My clients have excelled to seize opportunities to win the Charles Schwab Scholarship; an internship-then-job at Donna Karan, New York; and more. I'm grateful that I can support people to fulfill their Big Dreams,' says Tom Marcoux."

* * *

Now it's your turn.

Take a look at your experiences and efforts from the past. What have you learned? How do these learning experiences make you more valuable in the marketplace today?

Focus on these two questions:

- How can I take action today and build my personal brand?
- How can I stay aware of potential opportunities— even surprising ones?

Write your answers on paper or in your personal journal. While you're writing, encourage yourself by saying, *"Everything adds up"* and *"It all adds up to help me do better and better."*

(By the way, your personal brand is really a promise of your performance. How can people trust you to help them? Also, your personal brand is connected to the question: "What are you best known for?)

Imagine this: You are Uniquely Qualified

For those of us who have a spiritual path . . . you can realize that Higher Power has *guided you on this journey.* You have been prepared and now You are Uniquely Qualified for your next step—your next adventure.

Here's the Truth. It all comes down to your interpretation. Pick the Empowering Interpretation that every problem you've solved, every hurt you've endured has prepared you. You're now smarter, kinder, more empathetic and more prepared than before.

You are Uniquely Qualified to make this year better and better.

We learned how to take your experiences and view them in ways that make you more valuable to the marketplace.

Principle:
Take a long view to discover how your learning experiences can make you more valuable to the marketplace today.

Power Questions:
How can you take action today and build your personal brand? How can you stay aware of potential opportunities—even surprising ones?

Book Two / Topic #9

We now turn to this next article because happiness involves being fully alive and awake in the moment so you can create a *Magic Moment.*

Create a Magic Moment You'll Always Remember

The kiss shook me to the core of my being. I'm not kidding! This was my first kiss with my sweetie. It's 15 years later and we are soulmates. She believes in me and I believe in her! I'm so glad that I had the presence of mind to be fully alive for that moment.

We'll now cover what it takes to create a Magic Moment that you'll always remember. We'll use the C.A.N. process:

C – clear distractions
A – arrange your renewal
N – notice for 10 seconds

1. Clear distractions

Clear the distractions of fear and worry. Often, it feels hard to do that. It takes practice. For many of us, fear and worry arise when we're thinking of the future. Practice telling yourself, "I'm okay in this present moment." Here's another level of connecting to being "okay" in the present moment. Ask yourself, "Why am I okay in this present moment?" As author Noah St. John points out, asking "why" helps your brain shift into an empowered state.

I'll take this to another level: "Why am I *doing well* in this present moment?" Because I'm writing and feeling good about being helpful to readers. Because I'm taking deep breaths and I feel healthy and strong.

That's what you really want for clearing distractions from your mind—to get the "Because I am . . ." positive ideas to infuse your being.

2. Arrange your renewal

Many of us think of renewal as taking a walk in nature, seeing friends, and more. These forms are certainly vital.

Here is a different form of renewal, one that fills you with energy and helps you feel strong. I call it *"See-Your-Progress Renewal."*

For example, one of my former graduate students currently resides in Europe and wishes to gain a job in the USA. So I asked this former student via a Google chat:

"Do you currently have yourself on a 'job searching schedule'? That is, do you devote two hours a day (or more)? Do you have a log of efforts you do and the results you get?

...Do you have a contact management program that sends you email reminders so you keep up with all the details? ...

A *Progress Log* is quite useful to keep up your morale because it is your way of seeing your momentum and progress. A job search (like completing a feature film or a book) can feel like a long marathon.

A Progress Log notes:

Start, Stop, Duration of work,

Effort-Goals (tasks like phone calls, emails)

Result-Goals (number of phone interviews secured and completed)."

The Progress Log provides a different form of renewal: Hope.

We can look upon this hope as "renewal for your spirit."

Now it's your turn.

Will you set up a Progress Log for something important in your life?

3. Notice for 10 seconds

Researchers have noted that a person needs to pay attention to something positive for at least 10 seconds so that positive thing becomes *part of long term memory*. This is the crucial distinction about *"Create a Magic Moment You'll Always Remember"*: Write down for 10 seconds what positive things happened today.

Oprah Winfrey writes down positive details in her Gratitude Journal.

For years and to this day, every night for two and a half minutes, I write down positive details in my *Daily Journal of Victories and Blessings.*

I learned to do this because, when in college, I went to sleep sad nearly each night. Why? Because I had a to-do list that was *not* getting shorter. At night I was troubled with focusing on what I didn't get done during the day.

Ultimately, I rebelled against this and set up a healthy regimen of writing what I did well during the day (Victories) and the little joys of the day (Blessings).

Now it's your turn.

Will you use a small notebook and write down your Victories and Blessings of each day?

The truth is: Happy people know and *remember* what good things are in their lives.

To create a magic moment, you need to keep yourself strong and free of distractions.

To remember that magic moment, be sure to take 10 seconds and write it down in a *Daily Journal of Victories and Blessings.*

You'll feel better.
You'll get more done.
You'll enjoy life more.
My clients and I know this to be valuable and true.

We learned about the empowering question "Why am I doing well in this present moment?"

Principle:
Happy people know and *remember* what good things are in their lives.

Power Question:
Will you implement some personal version of a *Daily Journal of Victories and Blessings* in your life?

Book Two / Topic #10

I'm now sharing this next article because sometimes in our pursuit of happiness we get caught up in obsessing on just one thing. Instead, we need to realize that success and happiness possess three dimensions.

Use the Real Secret of Three-Dimensional Success

Imagine the man who arrived at success just in time to lose his marriage. Or the woman who took care of everyone but herself and died young. That's successful? I'm introducing "Success in 3 Dimensions."

Success in 3 Dimensions
- You feel great
- You're doing well in creating abundance
- Your health is terrific.

Having all three dimensions is essential to enjoying your successful life. When I say, "Doing well in creating abundance" I'm referring to a number of elements. Many of us truly want to enjoy what we do for a living. Further, we want to be well-compensated for it. Additionally, we'll find the idea of "abundance" to be useful. Abundance is about having a surplus—more than enough. If you have barely enough to pay rent and eat, that's NOT fun!

Many of us want cash to take a vacation, celebrate a loved one's birthday and more.

The question is: How can I have all three dimensions: feel great, create abundance and enjoy terrific health?

Here's the Real Secret of 3-Dimensional Success: It consists of three parts.
1) *"Life is about success, not perfection."* – Alan Weiss
2) *"It does not matter how slow you go as long as you do not stop."* – Confucius
3) *"Do something. It's Better than Zero."*
   – Tom Marcoux

1) "Life is about success, not perfection." – Alan Weiss

The problem with perfectionism is that it may shut down a person's desire and ability to perform a task. Fear sets in: if he or she can't get it right the first time, better to avoid the task. It is a vicious cycle of defeat.

If life is about success, then you can pay close attention and identify the vital elements of having a successful business, a successful relationship—and good health. As human beings, we're unlikely to do everything "perfectly," but we can focus on the *Most Important Things*.

For example, one of my clients walks 30 minutes a day and during that time talks with her boyfriend. Sure, perfection would include her doing vigorous weight training and running for two hours each day, but that does not match her lifestyle. So her body is not "perfect" in her own mind. But she does have a good romantic relationship; she's doing well at work and she gets appropriate sleep. She does *not* let her insecurities get in the way of enjoying life. She recognizes the *important elements* of a successful life.

Another way to view "success not perfection" is to declare: **Life is about taking effective action and making consistent progress.**

Now it's your turn.

Where are you allowing perfectionism to slow you down?

Are you spending your energy on "small things"? Are you neglecting the most important things that can improve your life?

2) "It does not matter how slow you go as long as you do not stop." – Confucius
Many of us have heard of the overnight success that took ten years.

My dad told me, "It takes fifteen years to be an overnight success", and it took me seventeen and a half years.
– Adrien Brody

The journey is important. Recently, I was teaching people how to go from zero connections to blog visitors from 141 countries. I realized that I had trained my whole life to teach that session and those people on that day.

Earlier in my business career, I worked for corporations doing work that had nothing to do with my best talents. Then, a decade later, I applied what I had learned to teaching graduate students at Stanford University.

All the experiences add up to make me more valuable in the marketplace today!

Now it's your turn.

How might you apply what you've learned over the years to making your life better and better?

3) "Do something. It's Better than Zero." – Tom Marcoux
Sometimes, the thing to do is study the situation or get more information. Sometimes the thing to do is take a break! When you return, you'll have a fresh perspective. For example, a client presented me with her notes for a blog article. At first, I was baffled. The notes were convoluted. I

took a break and returned and BAM! I could see the hidden thread that could run through the blog article.

My main point about "Do something. It's Better than Zero" is: *Take a step forward each day; they add up* . . . Two hundred words a day leads to a 52,000 word book (for example).

Laura Hillenbrand, the author of the bestselling books *Seabiscuit* and *Unbroken* endures Chronic Fatigue Syndrome. The article "The Unbreakable Laura Hillenbrand" notes: "Even the physical act of writing can occasionally stymie [Laura], as the room spins and her brain swims to find words in a cognitive haze. There have been weeks and months—indeed, sometimes years—when the mere effort to lift her hands and write has been all that she can muster."

Still, Laura takes a few steps forward each day. Let's notice that it all adds up: *Seabiscuit* has 399 pages and *Unbroken* includes 528 pages.

By the way, Laura's success is unusual. She does no talk shows and no in-person appearances promoting her books. Still, her books are bestsellers.

Now it's your turn.

What can you do today that is "better than zero"? How can you take some steps forward each day?

Remember, the people who truly enjoy life are making progress on all 3 *Dimensions of Success:*
- They feel great
- They're doing well in creating abundance
- Their health is terrific.

Remember "Life is about success, not perfection."

My added comment is: **Boldness makes progress. Precision makes sustainability.** By this I mean, you need to take a courageous step forward. You can refine your work as you go along so your work has lasting power.

Take some steps forward today.

We learned that feeling great, doing well in creating abundance and enhancing your health are involved in sustainable success and happiness.

Principle:
Boldness makes progress. Precision makes sustainability.

Power Question:
How can you do something positive and reap the benefits of "better than zero"?

Book Two / Topic #11

We now turn to this next article because feeling happy often involves feeling good after we've put ourselves in motion.

How to Get Inspired On Demand

"Today, I just don't feel inspired by what I'm writing," my client Norma said.

"I can help you with that," I assured her. Here's an important truth: To make a living at what you like doing, learn to shift your energy so you get to work immediately, regardless of your current mood.

"A professional is someone who can do his best work when he doesn't feel like it." – Alistair Cooke

We'll use the N.O.W. process:
N – notice where your heart is
O – open and walk forward
W – "write your story"

1. Notice where your heart is
Where is your heart? Are you sad? Is there a sad section of your work? Then work on that section.

If you feel listless and disconnected from the project you're working on, ask these questions:
- What is the real value of this project?
- Who does this project help?
- Where is the joy for me?

Often, when we lose the excitement for a project, it is because we're focusing on things that drain our energy.

Instead, notice where your heart is—that is, discover what about the project connects with your heart.

If you dig deep enough, you can find that heart connection . . . even if your task is shear drudgery. For example, someone I know procrastinated for 12 years about clearing out a big storage locker. But then one of his family members said she wanted to go to Avatarland (connected to James Cameron's feature film *Avatar*; the theme park opens as part of Walt Disney World in 2017). It was not saving money that got the guy into action. No, it was love for his family member!

2. Open and walk forward

As a professional writer, I do not pause for "writer's block." I choose to sit down and I write. No hesitation. I realize that I may not like what I'm writing for five minutes or so. Still, I just start writing anywhere I can in the project. If I do not have the perfect word, I put in a place holder "__MORE__."

When I say, "Open and walk forward," I mean that I begin and press on into today's session of work. I discover that, in the middle of doing the work, there are good moments to enjoy.

For example, when working on my graphic novel *Jack AngelSword*, I might find it becomes tedious to re-work and re-work some sections. I shift my focus to how much it means to me that Jack's logo on his chest represents his love for his god-daughter. Love is what empowers this story, and love inspires me!

On any project, I'm prepared to "push through the mud." There are certain parts of a project that I describe as "it's just work."

"Inspiration usually comes during work, rather than before it."
– Madeline L'Engle

Now it's your turn.

Where can you start so you can take a step forward with your project?

(This is connected to what I call *The Easy Part Start*. Start with an easy part and use the momentum to push through the difficult parts.)

An Important Part of *Open and Walk Forward*:

World-renowned Stanford University psychologist Carol Dweck emphasizes the **power of the "growth mindset"** over the timid "fixed mindset." The growth mindset accepts that mistakes, and sometimes "okay work," serve as stepping stones to better work. **It's all part of the process.** When you Open and Walk Forward, you hold the growth-mindset idea that today's work is all good practice for you to do better and better work.

So when I encourage you to *Open and Walk Forward*, I'm inviting you to get to work *even if you have some initial fear* that today's work may not be "good enough." If it's not, you can refine it by going back to it for another revision.

Otherwise, the next time you do similar work, you can do it better. Author Isaac Asimov (his name is on over 500 books!) was asked how he felt after turning in (to the publisher) his manuscript on Shakespeare. Isaac replied, "Like I'm ready to write a book on Shakespeare."

The point here is that even prolific writer Isaac Asimov acknowledged that the process of working today creates a better tomorrow because you become skilled at what you are doing. This process translates into better success in the future.

3. "Write your story"

Author Julia Cameron emphasizes that "original means you are the origin of the work." If you feel stuck, see if you can go deeper into your own story. The central idea for some of the best speeches in the world of the TED Conferences is "Be authentic." To be authentic, find something inside you that is true and that you want to express.

When I say, "Write your story," I mean that your art/project often works well when you are expressing a facet of what you know to be true.

Recently, one of my Facebook friends sent the question to her contacts: "What would you tell your younger self as inspiration? Say it in two words."

I first dismissed the question as being not useful. Just two words? I need at least a sentence! Then inspiration rose in my thoughts. Two words leapt into my mind: **Courageously Persist.**

That is good advice to myself and to you, my friend.

Develop courage. Expect that, in order to take your life to higher levels of success and happiness, you'll need to take calculated risks and . . . **Persist.**

Use the three methods of N.O.W.

N – notice where your heart is

O – open and walk forward

W – "write your story"

Hold yourself to a good standard. Do *not* give up when you might be in a low mood.

Take the low mood as *an invitation* to ask and answer these questions for yourself:

- What is the real value of this project?
- Who does this project help?
- Where is the joy for me?

And add this question: *How can I use this project to express some part of my heart and my truth?*

Find a way to express yourself.
It all adds up.

We learned about the process to "courageously persist."

Principle:
A low mood is an invitation for you to ask empowering questions for yourself.

Power Questions:
What is the real value of this project? Who does this project help? Where is the joy for you?

Book Two / Topic #12

I'm now sharing this next article because how we deal with our own anger has a huge impact on our daily experience of happiness and how much personal energy we have for exercise. It is possible to feel that someone wronged you and still shift your thoughts so you can move forward with your day.

How to Deal with Anger and Rise Up Stronger

Henry's father set him up so that Henry could not support his mother. Henry's mother was going into surgery, but his father would not tell Henry when the surgery was and forbid Henry from interacting with the doctor.

Then when Henry called, his father told his mother, "Marilyn, you aren't up for a visit are you?" Weak after surgery and from a culture that pushed women to give in to a husband's wishes, Henry's mother agreed to no visit. So Henry was forbidden to visit his mother on her difficult day.

At that moment, Henry felt bad and angry about how his father had become bitter and vindictive in his older years.

Many of us can relate to having to deal with a troublesome family member.

As we learn to adapt to the tough situations, it's important that we look beyond our anger and find ways to nurture ourselves and to get stronger. It's folly to try to change another person. It's better to develop more peace and calm in ourselves.

We'll use the N.E.W. process:

N – notice your part in the situation

E – examine the human behaviors

W – work out your personal action plan

1. Notice your part in the situation

The other person did you wrong, and you are justified in being angry. *Now what?*

I've learned the hard way that it's often necessary to pause, see what my own part is in the situation and then for me to come up with a plan for my *own* next actions. This is the path to feeling better.

I have a couple of elderly relatives who are just plain bitter and mean. They have Zero interest in listening or improving. I'm not going to change them.

The solution is: to recognize something about myself: I do NOT like to be at the mercy of someone else. So I need to plan with a focus on **what I am going to do the next time**.

When I have a plan and I personally take action, I feel empowered and hopeful.

Now it's your turn.

What can you do so that you can function better in the next tough situations you face?

2. Examine the human behaviors

I've learned that I can "skip being angry" sometimes by telling myself *"that's just a human being acting petty."* I do not expect human beings to always act from their better nature.

An important detail to examine is: What is my human vulnerability in this situation? If you're angry at someone, consider: Am I angry because I somehow let that other person get to me or hurt me?

Am I angry in part because: a) I fell for someone's lie? b) I allowed myself to get pushed into doing something that bothers me? c) I did not stand up for myself? or d) I did not stand up for someone else?

Make a plan of how you can live up to your own higher standards for your own behavior—for some possible future situation.

3. Work out your personal action plan

If you notice that you're on the edge, plan and take action to strengthen yourself. Get more sleep. Maybe trim some tasks off your schedule. We're not robots; we need rest and renewal.

Staying frazzled and tired can prolong and even worsen your feelings of anger. Instead, do what you need to do to make yourself stronger. Take a break. Get more sleep. Eat nutritious food. Drink more water to hydrate yourself. Devote time with a friend or family member you fully trust and who lifts your spirit.

"The weak can never forgive. Forgiveness is the attribute of the strong." – Mahatma Gandhi

What about forgiving yourself? Will you acknowledge that in the situation, you did the best you could with what you knew at the time?

Anger brought on by someone else's behavior and self-anger can often be related.

When you're angry, you'll do better in going beyond the simple "I'm angry at her/him." See how you can make a plan, take action, nurture yourself, and become stronger.

One of my favorite quotes is:

"Courage is not the absence of fear but rather the judgment that something is more important than fear." – Meg Cabot

I'll add: *Dealing well with anger is not about trying to change someone else. It's about making yourself stronger so you have more calm and focus beyond feelings of anger.*

Focus on:
"You're braver than you believe, and stronger than you seem, and smarter than you think." –A.A. Milne

To be smarter, expand your viewpoint. Take better care of yourself.

We learned about how being strong and skilled about anger involves self-reflection and planning your next, positive actions.

Principle:
See what might be your own part of a situation and then come up with a plan for your *own* next actions.

Power Questions:
Explore your own part in your anger. Are you angry because a) You fell for someone's lie? b) You allowed yourself to get pushed into doing something that bothers you? c) You did not stand up for yourself? or d) You did not stand up for someone else?

What can you plan for your next, positive actions?

Book Two / Bonus Topic #12a

I'm now sharing this next article because life has ups and downs. When we're in a dreaded slump, it may feel endless. The good news is that you can take action and rise to a better level.

You must take personal responsibility. You cannot change the circumstances, the seasons, or the wind, but you can change yourself. That is something you have charge of. – Jim Rohn

Jim Rohn talked about how winter comes every year. We do not change the seasons. I realized that *one needs to be skillful about dealing with winter* — or tough times.

When you have methods and strategies that you use, you can experience happy moments even when you're in winter. (Let's remember that happy moments yield more personal energy for you to devote to exercise.)

How You Can Bounce Back from a Slump

Maggie could feel it; she was in a dreaded slump. Her life felt "blah." She wasn't in the middle of a tragedy, but still she felt so tired, bored and — if she'd admit it — sad.

In a way, she reminded me of one of the most miserable people I had met. George was brilliant but uninvolved. He had no big joys because he simply didn't care about other people. That's a position that we're all advised to move beyond.

I've learned much from these three quotes:

1) "We must be willing to relinquish the life we planned so as to have the life that is waiting for us."

– Joseph Campbell

2) "The mystery of human existence lies not in just staying alive, but in finding something to live for."

– Fyodor Dostoyevsky

3) "The purpose of life is to contribute in some way to making things better." – Robert F. Kennedy

1) "We must be willing to relinquish the life we planned so as to have the life that is waiting for us."

– Joseph Campbell

Does your life feel bland? Too predictable? Look to see a clue that life has something new and different for you. This reminds me of a time I took up yoga. I was off on a new adventure. Every class I was trying something new.

2) "The mystery of human existence lies not in just staying alive, but in finding something to live for."

– Fyodor Dostoyevsky

Find something that gives you a smile. I know people who volunteer to take care of cats at the Humane Society, visit elderly people at a retirement home, and who write blogs because they want to support a small group of people scorned by a big group of people.

Find a way to give and life gives you feelings of joy and purpose.

3) "The purpose of life is to contribute in some way to making things better." – Robert F. Kennedy

Are you making something better? Even just a bit? Look for things you can improve. *Avoid* becoming adamant that other people change. Find out what you can do.

"I don't know what your destiny will be, but one thing I know: the only ones among you who will be really happy are those who will have sought and found how to serve." – Albert Schweitzer

I've learned something about getting out of a slump or being chronically miserable.

If you're miserable, your canvas is too small. You can be sad AND feel some purpose each day. It is an 'AND-Universe.' If we say that we are co-creating our life, and we have a paint brush in our hand . . . then don't limit the size of your canvas to just what you want. Imagine how you can *participate in life.*

On days when I have grieved the suicide of a dear friend, I have still taught college/graduate school classes. My day was not only about grief, it was also about serving others.

To bounce back from a slump, find some way to serve. Find some way to help someone. Just calling a friend and listening to her can brighten your day.

"Happiness is a perfume you cannot pour on others without getting some on yourself." – Ralph Waldo Emerson

Two weeks ago, my sweetheart said as I got out of her car, "Have a good day."

I replied, "Yes. I'll serve the students." And I did have a good day.

May you find a way to help others and warm your own heart.

Principle:
Find a way to give and life gives you feelings of joy and purpose.

Power Questions:

How can you give something and be helpful to someone else? How can you find someone to serve?

Now here are some guest articles related to happiness:

The reason I'm sharing this article by Mark Sanborn is: Mark invites us to focus on what is most important. For example, many us, when asked, would report our big reasons for dropping weight are to live pain free and avoid big health issues. Others would simply say that they want to appear more attractive. To be happy, it helps to focus on that which is most important.

8 Ideas to Make Your Life Better
by Mark Sanborn

1. You and I know how good we have become, but we don't have any idea of how good we could be.

What great projects are you undertaking in your business? In your life? Many people go through life driving with their dome lights on instead of their headlights. What you have become is important, but not nearly as important as what you can be.

2. Pursuing your potential is more important than achieving your goals.

It is satisfying to achieve your goals and objectives, but that's no proof that you are living up to your true capabilities. Keep experimenting and trying new things in the pursuit of your true potential.

3. Losers make excuses. Winners learn lessons.

Excuses don't teach you anything and keep you from making needed changes. Understanding why you failed will give you insights for needed changes.

4. Don't copy the crowd—learn from the leaders.

One of the quickest ways to become a leader is to learn from the leaders. Watch what the best are doing. Learn to do it. Then learn to do it even better.

5. Ask different questions to change your business or your life.

If you keep asking the same old questions you'll keep getting the same old answers. Rethink the situation and ask a different question.

I like what my friend Eric Chester said. He once reminded me that to keep growing you need a healthy form of skepticism that can be summed up in these words: "Answer your questions but question your answers."

6. Live by your values to achieve what is truly valuable.

A wise person once said, "The bad news is that you can't have it all. The good news is that when you know what's really important, you don't want it all anyway." Clearly identified values keep you on track and allow you to prioritize.

7. Focused attention beats brains and brute strength every time.

Continually ask yourself, "What gives me the biggest payback on my investment of time and energy?"

Focus on your mvp activities (most valuable and profitable). Spend 60-80% of every day on those mvp activities. That still leaves you with 20-40% of your time to deal with interruptions, crises and the unexpected.

8. You can't put more time in your life, but you can put more life into your time.

Do you "save time"? How much have you got saved up? Saving time is a myth. Time is a flow that cannot be interrupted. The best we can hope for is to use it wisely as it courses through our existence.

Put more life in your time by filling every moment with the richness of experience, learning, love and growth.

Mark Sanborn is the president of Sanborn & Associates, Inc., an idea lab for leadership development.

In addition to his experience leading at a local and national level, he has written or co-authored 8 books and is the author of more than two dozen videos and audio training programs on leadership, change, teamwork and customer service. He has presented over 2400 speeches and seminars in every state and a dozen countries.

Mark is a member of the prestigious Speakers Roundtable, 20 of the top speakers in the world today. Mark holds the Certified Speaking Professional (CSP) from the National Speakers Association and is a member of the Speaker Hall of Fame (CPAE).

The author of 8 books, Mark's book, *The Fred Factor: How Passion in Your Work and Life Can Turn the Ordinary Into the Extraordinary* was an international bestseller and has sold over 2 million copies. The sequel, *Fred. 2.0*, was released in March of 2013.

He is the leading authority on turning ordinary into

extraordinary and is in demand as a speaker, author and advisor to leaders.

Contact Mark at www.MarkSanborn.com

We learned about focusing on the most important aspects of life, success and happiness—in the above article. Working with such inspiration, I'll now provide you with my thoughts formed as a *principle* and *power question.*

Principle:
Focus on your values and discover amazing ways to fulfill your potential.

Power Questions:
What do you value most? Are you devoting significant attention, effort and time there? How can you shift your daily tasks so you are devoting time to what you value most?

* * * * * *

The reason I'm sharing this article by Noah St. John is: When you're clear about the power of an Empowering Daily Routine, you are energized to implement one in your life. Such an Empowering Daily Routine will likely support your Drop-Weight Plan.

Get an Empowering Daily Routine
by Noah St. John

What's the first thing you do when you get up in the morning?

Shrieking alarm clock... Check smartphone

Your first thought, "Oh brother, here we go again..."?

If this is how you START your day, what's the REST of your day going to look like?

Probably not so hot.

That's why Live Your DREAM Lesson #2 is to Get An Empowering Daily Routine.

What's an Empowering Daily Routine?

It's a ritual or set of habits that you do every day that, well, empowers you.

Why is it so important to have an Empowering Daily Routine?

1. Because life is tough enough without having to re-invent the wheel.

Many coaches, speakers, authors, healers, and mission-driven entrepreneurs don't have a blueprint or proven strategy for success.

Instead, they are basically flying by the seat of their pants every day—throwing spaghetti on the wall and seeing what sticks.

That is not a formula for success.

It's a recipe for disaster.

2. Because there's a big difference between an Empowering Daily Routine and a Disempowering Daily Routine.

We all follow daily routines.

Whether you get up at 6 am, 8 am, or 3 pm – whether you work from home or in an office – whether you drive to work, ride a bicycle, or walk from your bedroom to the kitchen – all human beings tend to follow routines.

The problem is that often these routines do not empower you – they DIS-empower you.

Of course, this happens gradually, over months, years, or decades.

But over time, we get stuck in a rut – caught in an endlessly-repeating cycle that keeps you stuck rather than sets you free.

3. Because structure gives you FREEDOM.

This is counter-intuitive, but when you follow a plan or blueprint, it doesn't hamper your creativity—it heightens it.

Many mission-driven entrepreneurs are also highly creative.

But there's a difference between being creative and being in chaos.

The irony is that the more structure you have in your day, the more you can actually free yourself to be more creative.

Why? Because rather than being distracted by every "shiny object" that comes along, you will be focused on your desired goal and have the confidence that comes from knowing you are working towards it.

If you don't have an Empowering Daily Routine, it's time to put one in place—both in your personal life as well as your business life.

The rewards of doing this simple act will astonish you.

Noah's Note: An Empowering Daily Routine gives you structure as it gives you freedom.

Noah St. John is a keynote speaker and best-selling author who is famous for inventing Afformations® and helping mission-driven entrepreneurs accelerate income, boost self-confidence, and enjoy financial freedom.

His sought-after advice is known as the "secret sauce" to overcome limiting beliefs and create lasting achievement.

According to Stephen Covey, author of *The 7 Habits of Highly Effective People:* "Noah St. John's work is about discovering within ourselves what we should have known all along—we are truly powerful beings with unlimited potential."

Harvey Mackay, author of *Swim with The Sharks Without Being Eaten Alive* says, "Noah speaks the language we all want to understand: how to make the most of your life and career."

Noah's dynamic and down-to-earth speaking style always gets high marks from audiences. As the leading authority on how to eliminate limiting beliefs, Noah delivers keynote speeches and mastermind programs that have been called "mandatory for anyone who wants to succeed in life and business."

He also appears frequently in the news worldwide, including ABC, NBC, CBS, Fox, The Hallmark Channel, National Public Radio, *Parade, Woman's Day, Los Angeles Business Journal, The Washington Post, Chicago Sun-Times, Selling Power,* Forbes.com, and The Huffington Post.

Fun fact: Noah once won an all-expenses-paid trip to Hawaii on the game show Concentration, where he missed winning a new car by three seconds. *(Note: He had not yet discovered the Power Habits® Formula.)*

Get the first chapter of Noah's latest bestseller AFFORMATIONS®: The Miracle of Positive Self-Talk FREE at www.NoahStJohn.com

We learned about the Empowering Daily Routine in the above article. Working with inspiration from the above article, I'll now provide you with my thoughts formed as a *principle* and *power question.*

Principle:

Set an Empowering Daily Routine and enjoy having more energy to apply to your Drop-Weight Plan.

Power Question:

What one daily routine can really raise the level of your game (higher success, more happiness)?

[When you're happier, you have more energy for your Drop-Weight Plan.]

* * * * * *

The reason I'm sharing this next article by Craig Harrison is: *happiness often involves focusing on the best and letting go of "the good."* Commitment actually frees you to experience passion and joy. Many years ago, I wrote about what I called "freedom through commitment." Pick what you're committed to and drop what you have lukewarm feelings for.

Are You Committed or Just Involved?
by Craig Harrison

Are you working a job or building a career? Are you punching a time clock or chiseling a body of work, a day at a time. Perhaps you have heard about the two laborers setting bricks at a construction site. When asked, one said he was building a wall, while the other boasted he was constructing the Sistine Chapel. What is the big picture? Are you a bystander or are you in the game? It's time you commit.

If you're unclear on the difference between being involved vs. committed, consider your last ham and egg breakfast. The chicken was involved. The pig...committed. (Have you heard an oeuf already?) Your career is too important not to be committed to it. Committed fruit-pickers don't quit once the low hanging fruit's been picked. They know where the best fruit is to be gotten. They commit to climb high and reach far out on the branches!

The Long And Winding Road
Successful professionals think longer term. Lay your own foundation for the long haul. Do you look around the bend and anticipate what's to come? Do you create plans in terms of decades and years, rather than months and days? Invest

in yourself and plan for the marathon ahead.

Many Moves Ahead

Are you saving or just spending? Are you preparing for rainy days and down times, for hurricanes and floods? Are you building a support system and continuing to educate yourself in your chosen field and beyond? Are you reading *Transaction World* cover to cover? Cover all bases by staying ahead of the field. Chess masters play many moves ahead. It's not enough to show up for each match. Play to win! This year, commit to taking a new class, read cutting edge books on subjects of relevance to your field, attend the annual ETA Meeting and Expo, engage a sales or professional coach, or otherwise commit yourself to excel in the new year.

Motivate From Within

Committing to be the best means being your best. Excellence starts within. I can egg you on to bring home the bacon but ultimately it's the fire within you that will fuel your success. With this column I thee commit to greatness this year! Game on!

Craig Harrison's ExpressionsOfExcellence.com provides sales and service solutions for organizations and communication and leadership development for individuals. Based in the San Francisco Bay Area, Craig is a speaker, trainer, author, consultant, coach and storyteller and an active leader in the National Speakers Association, Toastmasters International and National Storytelling Network

* Download Craig's free Quick Start Guide to finding the best Toastmasters club for you!

www.ExpressionsOfExcellence.com/Toastmasters/QuickS

tartGuide_Toastmasters.pdf

We learned about deciding to be committed and achieving on the highest levels.. Working with this inspiration, I'll now provide you with a *principle* and *power question*.

Principle:
Focus on preparation and "many moves ahead."

Power Questions:
What most important things are coming up for you? How can you prepare and then be at your best? What resources will you use? Will you read top books, listen to audio books, engage a coach or rehearse?

* * * * * *

The reason I'm sharing this next article by Dr. Elayne Savage is: To create true and sustained happiness, we need to face our blind spots. In this process, we grow and become stronger.

Blind Spots—Those Unacceptable Parts of Ourselves
by Elayne Savage, PhD

I've been thinking a lot about blind spots lately. Mine and other peoples.

Blind spots are those traits about ourselves we just don't see, although other folks do.

My favorite quote about blind spots is from the 2001 movie *Yi Yi:*

"I can't see what you see and you can't see what I see. How can we know more than half the truth?"

Yi Yi is the family's wise young son who takes photos of the backs of people's heads. "You couldn't see it," he says, "so I showed you."

We soon discover in the movie, what people cannot see is what they choose not to see. Yi Yi's mission is to take pictures of their pain.

And it is the same with our own blind spots. Where does this lack of ability to "see" ourselves come from?

Those Submerged Parts of Yourself
Often, we are unable to acknowledge certain aspects of ourselves. Parts of our personalities stay hidden from us because they are not acceptable to us. This is what Carl Jung called *the shadow*—the dark part, the part we don't want to know about ourselves, and wish wasn't there.

How does this come about? In childhood we begin to notice we bring on someone's displeasure by displaying certain emotions or behaviors or ideas or attitudes. Sometimes these messages are cultural or gender-connected.

Because we sensed these emotions or actions were unacceptable to others, we interpreted this as "bad," so we submerged them.

In other words, we forget to look in the mirror and we lose our authentic self somewhere along the way.

Robert Johnson, in *Owning Your Own Shadow*, reminds us that these "refused and unacceptable characteristics do not go away; they only collect in the dark corners of our personality."

They especially begin to seep out when we judge or criticize others. We often cannot tolerate in others the very same traits we can't stand about ourselves.

Through a process called *projection*, we mistakenly imagine these unacceptable traits exist in the other person when we cannot acknowledge them in ourselves. These traits are most likely our blind spots.

A woman I know says, "If we can't own our own stuff, we try to give it away to someone else. In a way, projection protects us from ourselves by spreading the garbage around."

Let's Talk About Projection

Our "blind spots" can certainly affect relationships with other people. Traits you project onto others might include your sadness, your anger, your tendency to be snarky or cynical or patronizing or manipulative or flirtatious or competitive or controlling.

Might these be *your* own characteristics? Your own blind spots?

What can *you* add to this list?

Projection often involves blaming the other person for our own limitations. And most of us are all too aware that blame creates resentment and resentment takes up so much space in relationships there is no room for connection and intimacy.

Those Rejected Parts of Yourself

Robert Johnson says some of these hidden characteristics are "pure gold"—but we end up rejecting these parts of ourselves because they were unwelcome to our family or society.

Recognizing these disavowed parts and owning your shadow side as well as your more desirable features is an important part along the road of getting to know yourself. Intimacy with yourself is the key to acquiring the capacity for intimacy with another person..

By getting to know yourself, you can identify and do something about your needs for closeness and distance and not have to be constantly refereeing that internal conflict.

What about you? What might *your* shadow side be? Where does it come from and why did you have a need to hide it away? Are you able to identify it in yourself or do you deal with it through spotting it in other people? How often does this happen in your personal relationships? In the workplace?

How Can You Change Something If You Can't See It?

It's pretty hard to change something if you are not even aware of it.

By recognizing, identifying and becoming an objective observer, you can put yourself in a position to make some choices about how you want to "be" in relationships.

When you begin to notice that you are becoming judgmental of someone or that you simply can't stand them, it just might be you are recognizing your own behavior! This act of noticing is a great way to get to know yourself.

The best way to change something is to notice it. Yep. It's really difficult to do something differently if you can't see it.

Why not practice walking alongside yourself, noticing your thoughts and feelings and reactions. Then decide if you want to keep walking down the same path or if you want to go back to the fork in the road and try out another path.

Will the Real You Please Stand Up?

Next, become aware of how rejection plays a role here—especially judgments and criticism. By recognizing signs of rejection and noticing how you react to it, you're taking the first steps in giving yourself some distance and the opportunity to do something differently.

Recognizing the disavowed parts, the dark side, leaves less room for critical judgment of others and of yourself as well. Owning your shadow side as well as your more desirable features is an important part of the road to self-acceptance—to wholeness.

There's a lot of room in there for all the parts to coexist. Why not encourage them to befriend each other? Each part could teach the others quite a few things. They all have information to share, but you'll find some of them are more talkative than others. Try getting to know them.

What are *Your* Blind Spots?

Of course if they really are blind spots, you may answer, "I don't know. I don't see any." Often, however, the submerged traits are floating just below the surface and with a little attention can become accessible.

A good analogy of blind spots of course is about driving a car: The standard blind spot analogy typically describes an area immediately outside your own vehicle, yet close enough so that you cannot see objects in these areas by using your side mirrors alone.

Good ideas for cars and relationships: Look out for potential dangers and don't forget to look in your mirror or even turn your head and look around you!

Excerpted from *Don't Take It Personally! The Art of Dealing with Rejection* and *Breathing Room—Creating Space to Be a Couple*

Dr. Elayne Savage, The Queen of Rejection®, is a skillful communication coach and internationally respected expert on how not to take rejection and disappointment so personally.

Elayne has over twenty-five years in coaching, consulting, and clinical experience. She holds a Ph.D. in Family Psychology.

A professional member of the National Speakers Association, she is a sought-after workshop leader, trainer, and consultant for a broad range of clients. An expert on criticism and rejection, cultural diversity, resilience, and work and family relationships. Elayne educates, inspires and challenges audiences.

Elayne is the author of two internationally acclaimed books published in 9 languages: *Don't Take It Personally! The Art of Dealing with Rejection* (New Harbinger; M.J. Fine Publications; iUniverse) and *Breathing Room—Creating Space to Be a Couple* (New Harbinger Publications; iUniverse.)

Her popular blog,
www.TipsFromTheQueenOfRejection.com

focuses on rejection, fear of rejection and self-acceptance. She is based in the San Francisco Bay Area.

We learned "the best way to change something is to notice it" in the above article. Working with such inspiration, I'll now provide you with a *principle* and *power questions.*

Principle:
Notice your thoughts and feelings and then decide how you might address them to improve your life.

Power Questions:
What are your first thoughts about a possible "rejected part of yourself"? How might you be kind to yourself as you take action to become more aware and stronger?

* * * * * *

The reason I'm sharing the next article by Dr. Willie Jolley is: Many of us discover our happiest moments when we take appropriate risks, and we feel enthusiastic while we stretch and grow.

[To continue with a theme of this book: create more happy moments and you'll have more personal energy to devote to your Drop-Weight Plan.]

Dr. Willie Jolley's Thought of the Day: How I Overcame My Fear of Quitting My Job!

a lightly edited transcript
of a video by Dr. Willie Jolley

I had recently shared a video online about my experience of starting my company on June the First, 1991. I shared with my staff what set me up to make that decision to leave my job. I was working at a good government job, and I hated it.

I hated it because the people were so negative. They were toxic. Every time I would come up with a new idea and say, "Hey, let's try this" – they replied, "No. That's not going to work."

"How about this?" I'd ask.

"No. That's not going to work."

Every time I would try something new, they would cut me off at the knees. I got discouraged. In fact, some days, I had to go to my mother's house and lay down at lunchtime because I was so sick.

But one day, after working all year, not having a break, not having any vacation or time off, I went to my boss. I said, "A friend of mine has offered my wife and me an opportunity to go with them to their vacation spot for a few days—just to relax. I'd like to do that. So I'd like to take a couple of days off."

She said, "No."

"But, but—I just want to take a few days off because I worked all year," I continued.

"You have sick leave but you don't have any annual leave. It's not part of your job package."

I said, "Really? Come on, can I use my sick leave?"

"No. You have to call in everyday for your sick leave. Day by day. No," she said.

I was crushed. But I made up my mind as to what I would do. So everyday, I'd get up and I would call and say that I was sick. But I was sick; I was mentally sick.

I came back after that vacation and I told my boss: "I realize that this job is not a good fit for me. And I need to leave."

And I left. I remember the day, May 31st. I walked out of there and my co-workers laughed at me and said, "You'll be back! You fool. You're leaving your good government job to go become a speaker. Hah! You're gonna starve."

In fact, they took me to lunch on my last day. They said, "You need every free meal you can get."

But the next day, June 1st, a Saturday, I set up my little company with a card table, a legal pad, phone book and a touch-tone phone. But I had one other thing: I had a dream. And I set out on that dream June the First, 1991.

I'm grateful that in these years that have gone by, I have been inducted into the Speaker Hall of Fame, named one of the Top Five Speakers. I had bestselling books, a television show, a radio show. I've literally traveled the world and I have had a ball making a difference.

And I told my co-workers I would be back...and I did

come back…three years later…as their keynote speaker! And when I came back I was paid a fee for an hour that was three times more than what I had been making for working all week!

There are some things that I've learned in this process. One, sometimes you got to take a stand. I love this little quote: "As long as you stand up, no one can ride your back." The other is that it truly is liberating to live your dreams. Some people get mad and want to get even, but I didn't want to get even…I made up my mind to Get Ahead, because I figured out that massive success truly is the best revenge!

So don't get mad so you can just get even. Get up and get ahead! Stand up. Stand up for your dreams, make a decision and have the courage to step out and make it happen!

Another thing I've learned is this: That which is before you and that which is behind you can never compare with that which God has placed within you. There is something special inside you. You were born with greatness—the seeds of greatness—inside you. But you've got to be willing to water, fertilize and develop those seeds. And make the most of the gifts that God has given you.

So I'm encouraging you to live your dreams. That's my thought of the day. Sometimes, you have to make a decision. And you CAN if you think you can.

This is Dr. Willie Jolley. Have a great day. God bless you.

Dr. Willie Jolley, CPAE, CSP

There are many inspirational/motivational speakers, and then there is the one, the only, the incomparable Dr. Willie Jolley. He is a Hall of Fame Speaker, an Award-Winning Singer, a Best-Selling Author and a National Television & Radio Personality. The Business Ad Hoc Committee recently tabbed him as "The #1 Inspirational Speaker/Singer in America" and he is was invited to replace the legendary Zig Ziglar on the national Get Motivated Seminars Tour across America.

Dr. Willie Jolley has achieved remarkable heights in the speaking industry, having come from humble beginnings of being a fired singer (who was replaced by a karaoke machine!). He has gone on to be named "One of the Outstanding Five Speakers in the World" & "Inspirational/Motivational Speaker of The Year" by the 175,000 members of Toastmasters International. He has been inducted into the prestigious Speaker Hall of Fame as well as achieving the distinction of Certified Speaker Professional by the National Speakers Association. In addition, he is also the recipient of the Ron Brown Distinguished Leadership Award and the African American Chamber of Commerce DC Business Leadership Award.

Dr. Willie Jolley uses his public platform to pursue his mission of empowering and encouraging people to rise above their circumstances and maximize their God given potential! Many know him as the speaker Ford Motors called on in 2006 when they were on the brink of bankruptcy, and he worked with them in 2006, 2007 and 2008, and in 2009 they were able to reject a government bailout and go on to Billion Dollar profits.

He is the author of several international best-selling books including *It Only Takes A Minute To Change Your Life, A Setback Is A Setup For A Comeback, Turn Setbacks Into Greenbacks* and *An Attitude of Excellence,* which was endorsed by Dr. Stephen Covey. No matter the venue, from his exciting television appearances to his #1 Rated SiriusXM radio show, to corporate audiences like Wal-Mart, Ford, GM, Comcast, Verizon, Marriott or The Million Dollar Round

Table … Dr. Willie Jolley keeps it moving with high energy and enthusiasm, as he delivers nuggets on how every person can live a better life, one day at a time!
www.williejolley.com
Office: (202) 723-8863

We learned about taking an appropriate risk and bringing new blessings into one's life. Working with inspiration from the above article, I'll now provide you with my thoughts formed as a *principle* and *power question*.

Principle:
Take an appropriate risk and raise your life to a wonderful level.

Power Questions:
Is there an appropriate risk that can truly enhance your life? What are your willing to do to prepare and take action to make your life so much better?

* * * * * *

The reason I'm sharing this article by Coco of *Light by Coco* is: Research demonstrates that much unhappiness is caused by money troubles. If you're miserable due to misguided spending habits, you can feel so drained that you turn to food for comfort.

I've learned much about saving and being good with money budgets by watching my father's errors. I saw the results he had, and I decided that I wanted something different and better. For example, one year a commercial truck backed into my father's car, smashing it. He received a settlement from the insurance company. He said, "Let's go on a family vacation." I said, "I can't get away from work at this time. How about you place it in a CD (certificate of deposit at the bank). You could renew the CD every month until we can take the vacation."

My father never placed the money in a CD at the bank. Instead, he just bought stuff—a little of this and a little of that. And my family never went on that vacation.

So it means a lot to me that my former college student Coco is now sharing her effective spending strategies here:

How I Changed My Spending Habits
a lightly edited transcript of a video
by Coco of *Light By Coco*

When I started decluttering, I realized that the only way I could stay clutter free was to change the way things were coming in. I also wanted to save more money for the things that were truly important to me. So I had to change my spending habits. These are some tips that helped me stay focused in creating my new habit of not buying as much as before:

1. START SAVING UP: Every day or week you go without shopping, put a small amount of money aside. When you are focused on saving up for something bigger and more important, it's easier to resist small impulse purchases.

2. ONE IN, ONE OUT RULE: For every object that comes in, something has to be donated or sold. If you have to get rid of something you already own, you'll probably think a little harder about whether you really want the item in the store. It's also a great way to stop way too much clutter from building up in your space.

3. RE-THINK SALES: Get out of the habit of thinking that something is worth buying just because it's on sale. Ask yourself whether it would be worth buying if it weren't on sale. A lot of stores go with a "this weekend only sale" strategy; don't fall for it. There will be another sale, another weekend when you actually need something new.

4. GET RID OF TEMPTATION: When you don't receive catalogues in the mail or weekly emails from stores you lessen the prompts that create that "I need something new" itch. Unsubscribe!

5. SHOP YOUR CLOSET: Try out new combos at home, right from your own closet. Try on six shirts at once, go as avant-garde as you like, no one is watching and you might end up finding a great new outfit.

6. JUST DON'T GO: Staying away from physical as well as online stores reduces the urge for impulse purchases. If you're not there, you can't buy anything.

7. TIME DELAY: Put the item you're thinking of buying on hold and leave the store. If you still want it after a couple of hours pass, then go get it. Or you can walk around in the store with the item you're interested in for a while. The time delay reduces the chance of an impulse purchase. Same goes

for online shopping: put everything you'd like in your basket. Just don't checkout until another time (I'm willing to bet the total price will be enough to make you change your mind.)

8. LEAVE YOUR ENABLER AT HOME: We talking about that friend who says, "Yes, get it. It looks totally amazing!" or "It's on sale; you should get it now." You don't have to go shopping alone. Just make sure you bring a more critical friend—someone who real-talks you by asking questions like "Do you really need another pair of suede boots?" Not as fun, but definitely effective.

9. DITCH THE PLASTIC: This is more applicable to some people than others. But if you stick to cash, you have a finite amount of money before you have to run to an ATM. Seeing your money physically disappear can also be an incentive to slow down.

10. BE PICKY: Make sure you have a reason as to why you are buying something. Go shopping with a list. This action reminds you why you came to the store in the first place. Before checking out, go over the list and make sure you're not getting anything that's not on it. Also, make sure the things you are buying are pretty close to perfect. If you're looking for a new blazer, make sure it's exactly what you're looking for. Does it fit right? What color are the buttons? What material is it? Don't rush and don't settle.

11. PLAY PRETEND: Now depending on how well you have your shopping habits under control, this tip can either help you or tempt you. I go on websites like Polyvore or Pinterest and play virtual dress up by combining clothes and collecting images which I don't have to purchase. I like Pinterest because it lets me express my style without spending any money. Time with Pinterest helps me to avoid cluttering up my life.

12. WHY? Figure out why you are shopping and address the issue. Maybe you're insecure or filling a void. Or you're just plain bored!

13. RETURN IT: If you do end up buying something and feel remorse, don't sweat it! Most items can be returned unopened with tags still attached. Just make sure that if you do feel buyer's remorse, you actually go back and return it. Don't be tempted to buy something else when returning to the store! I have the habit of asking a store clerk about the return policy. If the return policy is strict, the threshold for buying something is even higher. And I am less likely to buy something unless I'm 100% sure.

14. LEAVE FREEBIES BE: This is more of a way to stop clutter creep but, don't accept freebies! Free t-shirt, no. Buy five body lotions and get a free tote, nope. Free key chains at a convention, no. If you wouldn't buy it, leave it. It will only clutter up your house.

Light by Coco is a lifestyle blog which focuses on applying living light to every aspect of life. When Coco started paring down her belongings in 2011 to make a pending move easier, she realized that the lack of stuff was the change she didn't know she needed.

After seeing how living with less translated so well into all aspects of her life, she decided to create a YouTube channel and blog to share her experiences. With her blog, Coco aims to inspire people to make positive changes in their lives and in turn create a more conscious consumer.

We learned about effective spending habits in the above article. Working with such inspiration, I'll now provide you with my thoughts formed as a *principle* and *power question.*

Principle:

Use strategy in how you spend money and be sure to save a significant portion of each check that comes in.

Power Question:

What would really brighten your life—if you saved money for it each month?

* * * * * *

We now turn to this next article by Chris Shelton because it's important to listen to the voice of intuition for your happiness and more.

Find Your Footing Before You Fall
by Chris Shelton

As my daughter screamed and slipped over the cliff's edge, an icy stillness washed over me. If I could just stay present and calm, I knew I could save my child. All I needed was one more miracle.

After everything that happened that day what I remember most is the feeling of peace. What could have been the worst day of my life was transformed into my best.

Pinnacles National Park is just outside of San Jose, California. The mountainous area is a popular place for camping and hiking. But that hot summer afternoon no one was there except me, my wife and four children. It was as if the rest of the world was quiet and still; like all the elements – earth, water, metal, wood and fire – were balanced and singing in silent harmony.

My family, on the other hand, was loud and active. We were celebrating Sabreena's last few days at home before she left for college. She was 18, happy and dressed like the rest of us – t-shirt, shorts, flip-flops. None of us had water or a flashlight as we walked along the hiking path leading to the park's most famous cave.

As we left the bright clearing of the picnic area into the cool shade of the ancient oaks, California condors, a kind of vulture, soared above us. I remember the sound of my children's laughter bouncing off the trees and rocks as they raced ahead, my wife chasing after them.

And then Sabreena vanished.

A scream and the sounds of rock falling into space.

My baby girl, my eldest daughter, had somehow slipped into a talus cave, an opening between two giant boulders. Each boulder was as tall as a 10-storey building! Every time Sabreena squirmed to free herself, the ancient rocks tightened their squeeze and pulled her further into the darkness and away from me.

With my wife and other children out of sight and no longer within earshot, it was just me and my daughter and the gnawing anxiety that what was happening was about to get much, much worse.

Sabreena was sobbing and begging that I not leave her. Each time she lifted her hand to grab mine, she slid deeper into the jagged crevice. Pebbles and gravel rolled out from under her. I never heard one of those rocks hit the cave floor.

If Sabreena fell, how far would she fall?

I anchored my feet and body so I could pull her up with all my might. I'm a big guy who's been kickboxing and studying martial arts since I was a kid; pulling my 110-lbs daughter to safety was not going to be a problem.

"If you pull her, she will die."

A crystal clear voice from within.

I knew the voice. It had saved my life 20 years ago. A near-fatal heart attack had been transformed into a near-death-experience, leaving me with memories of unconditional peace, acceptance and love.

Doctors called my recovery from heart failure a miracle; a return to wellness they could not understand or explain.

And here was the same voice that had guided me back to life promising me it could save my daughter's life, if I chose peaceful intuition over brute-force instinct.

"If you pull her, she will die.

Let Sabreena find her footing."

Imagine your most joyful moment, best meditation, prettiest sunset. Now imagine feeling those positive emotions while watching your child dangle from a cliff's edge. Seems wrong, doesn't it? Yet in the moment my daughter needed me most—she needed me to save her life— I was fully present and peaceful.

I knew that if Sabreena fell, I would fall with her. There was no way my daughter was going to fall from that height alone.

Crawling along that jagged ledge with vultures above me and Sabreena's whimpered cries below me, I was in the most peaceful place I could ever imagine. Dying—or living— didn't matter; I could accept whatever happened. From that pure peaceful place came the wisdom to act effectively and without panic.

I reached down, Sabreena grabbed my arm and started regaining her footing. She was literally walking up the side of the boulder.

Every time I was tempted to rush the process and pull her up, my inner voice warned, "This looks like the way, but it is not the way."

"If you pull her, she will die."

After what seemed like an eternity, Sabreena was safe and above ground.

"I almost died down there, didn't I?" she asked in a quiet, startled voice.

A day that started out as a celebration of Sabreena's new life at college ended as a near-death experience for both of us.

What could have been a tragic and brutal accident was in fact a blessing that continues to enrich and shape my life. My relationship with my daughter was transformed; today we both know what unconditional love feels like.

The indescribable peace of pure surrender, pure acceptance has stayed with me. I believe that peacefulness is Universal Intelligence, God, Source—whatever word you use to describe the sweet mystery of life.

Happily, you don't have to fall off a cliff and into a cave to achieve enlightenment!

Today my commitment to Qigong, self-healing through gentle breaths and gentle movements—think "yoga" but easier and more powerful—is richer and deeper. When clients leave my office free from pain and fear, I believe they've accessed their own inner healing, their own inner voice that knows the way back to perfect safety, well-being and joy.

The voice that saved me and my daughter is within you.

Listen deeply, move mindfully, breathe lovingly.

You'll pull yourself out of the crevice and off the ledge.

When you tune in to your inner wisdom, you do fall... you fall in love with life.

Chris Shelton is a certified Qigong practitioner and teacher. He's studied with some of China's most revered traditional Chinese medicine masters. As a teenager Chris was almost paralyzed by a martial-arts back injury. He attributes his full recovery to Qigong. Today Chris is an award-winning martial arts fighter, author of two books about Qigong, and a professional speaker and workshop leader. Chris has taught self-healing techniques to at-risk youth, professional fighters, paraplegics and celebrities looking for deeper meaning in their lives. In the summer of 2015 Chris led a stadium-wide demonstration of Qigong to thousands of attendees at the Special Olympics Opening Ceremonies in Los Angeles. Chris belly laughs at least 11 times a day and can be found chasing after his "herd of turtles," his family, in San Jose, California. For downloads about using Qigong to improve your health without pain, surgery or drugs, visit

http://www.qigongforselfrefinement.com/book/

Since Chris Shelton spoke of Qigong, here is his description of this ancient tradition:

"Qigong is an ancient tradition of short meditations and simple physical exercises. Move your hand here, imagine a color, say a sound. The techniques are deceptively simple yet produce profound results in the realm of mind-body-spirit health. Think of Qigong as the "new yoga" for people wanting to connect with their intuitive wisdom. Qigong is suitable for everyone (young, old, athletic, immobile) because the exercises are gentle and slow, and can be done standing, sitting or laying down. Rooted in traditional Chinese medicine, Qigong has been a healthcare secret for centuries in China. Whether working with a professional Qigong practitioner or practicing independently, people experience a greater sense of peace and joy within minutes. For people living in chronic pain, Qigong has proven to offer immediate, long-lasting relief. Western medicine is slowly adopting Qigong practices as more and more reports emerge from the East about patients experiencing spontaneous recoveries without surgery or drugs."

* * * * * *

The reason I'm sharing this next article by Randy Gage is: *happiness often involves a shift in perspective.* When we're living a life with feelings of enthusiasm, sometimes a project will fail to give us our preferred results. We might call the project a failure. However, there is much to harvest from a so-called failure.

Refuse to Lose

A lightly edited transcript of a video
by Randy Gage

You ever see on Facebook: Who was this person? Ran for Congress—Lost, Ran for this—Lost, Ran for that—Lost, Had a nervous breakdown . . . It's twenty things in row. And you find out that it's Abraham Lincoln.

A similar thing is with Walt Disney who went bankrupt many times before reaching success with Disneyland, Walt Disney World, the studio and all of that.

I want to talk this week about overcoming failure. I'm really qualified to talk about that because I have failed so many times.

When Steve Jobs passed away, we saw that he was a guy born out of wedlock and he didn't have a college degree. He was thrown out of his company, Apple. Then, look at what a difference Steve Jobs made in the end and how many lives he touched in the world.

When I look at my life and the things that I have been through: first business through fifth business failing; business seized by the I.R.S. and auctioned off for taxes. I got shot in a robbery. I think of all these failures and traumatic experiences I've had; and I say that I wouldn't change anything in my life because I have used obstacles, challenges, failures and setbacks to move forward.

And you can do the same thing. But there are just a couple of things you need to keep in mind:

First, you've got to understand that obstacles can be stepping stones to achievement. They can allow you to develop the strength of character, gain new skills, and make changes in your course.

Second, if you recognize obstacles as wake-up calls and learn what you need to learn, you learn the lesson the universe is trying to tell you. Otherwise, the universe is going to send the lesson to you again and again—like I had to get it many times until I thought, "Maybe I can learn this lesson and then I can move on to the next course."

Look for the lesson.

Finally, refuse to lose. You just recognize that failure is part of the success process. We test, track, modify and change. And we move forward. *If you don't give up, you can always win.*

Make that a mantra to yourself: *Refuse to lose*

Additional Lesson: Find people who have done successfully what you want to do, and model those people. Follow them for guidance. Seek them for mentorship. Look for successful people and follow the patterns that they have developed. I would sum up the lesson as *Stop taking financial advice from broke people*. Don't talk to Uncle Herbie who tried something 20 years ago or other family members who are not really successful. These are not the people you talk to. If you're like I was when I started out and I didn't have family or friends who were really successful, then you use the videos, DVDs, and books of millionaires and billionaires.

Randy Gage is the author of nine books, including the *New York Times* bestseller, *Risky Is the New Safe*. He has spoken in 48 U.S. States, all Canadian provinces and 48 other countries, to more than 2 million people. He was listed in the "Who's Hot" article for *Speaker Magazine* and in 2013 was inducted into the Speakers Hall of Fame.

www.RandyGage.com

Prosperity TV at http://www.youtube.com/randygage

We learned that "obstacles can be used as stepping stones to achievement" in the above article. Working with such inspiration, I'll now provide you with a *principle* and *power question*.

Principle:

We do not fail if we use what we learn to continue to test, modify, change and improve what we're doing.

Power Question:

How can you apply what you learn so you can test, modify and improve what you're doing?

BOOK THREE:
Excel with More Time
(Have More Time to Exercise when You Earn More AND Work Less)

As the Caltrain arrived in San Francisco, I stood near the door of the first car. I was poised to quickly exit the train because in this particular semester the lecture hall was significantly further from the train station. In essence, I had a new problem: My commute time had doubled. So it was more time invested at the same rate of earning. At this point in my career, I was thinking that I needed to earn more money. Would I teach more classes, or could I think of other ways to create streams of income?

Many of us are so pressed by work hours and family obligations that we *cannot* even imagine devoting more time to exercise and other health-enhancing activities.

In answer to that dilemma, I will now share strategies so that you can *Earn More and Work Less.*

My intention is to take a holistic approach to dropping

weight. Further, I am *avoiding* repeating the same material found in many weight loss books.

Many of us who read weight loss books just nod our heads. We even shake our heads and say, "Oh, that's nice — if my fulltime job was exercising and modeling." Since most of us will not have that focus, I'm writing about an important part of your Drop-Weight Plan: to make space in your schedule to exercise.

Truly, if you earned more, *you could cut back* some of your work hours and devote them to health-enhancing activities.

Toward that end, we'll use the E.A.R.N.M.O.R.E. process:

E – enact leadership
A – ask better questions
R – respect to inspect
N – neutralize "occupational hobbies"
M – make good budget decisions (face the pain)
O – open to new systems
R – raise your fees
E – empower hiring and delegating

1. Enact leadership
To have more time for your exercise, consider the power over your schedule you can have when you become a leader of projects.

I often share with my audiences this idea:
You can be paid by the hour or . . .
you can be "paid by leadership."

By "paid by leadership," I mean that you lead projects and let other people accomplish the work while you're not even in the room.

Getting paid by leadership is about you *not* doing all the

work. There is *no* ceiling in terms of your earning power when you lead projects.

In order to lead well, we learn to ask better questions . . .

2. Ask better questions

A first step to earning more is to ask better questions. Upon reflection, we realize that we deal with two forms of questions: *Draining Questions* and *Empowering Questions*.

"Why does this always happen to me?" is a Draining Question.

"How can I use this to make me stronger and smarter?" is an Empowering Question.

Someone I know was rather miserable for a time and then chose to step out of my life. If I met this person tomorrow, I'd have a question: "Did you find someone to serve?"

"I don't know what your destiny will be, but one thing I know: the only ones among you who will be really happy are those who will have sought and found how to serve." – Albert Schweitzer

Yesterday, just before I exited the family car to get on a train, my sweetheart said to me, "Have a good day at work."

"I'll serve the students," I replied. And in saying this, I acknowledged my joy at being helpful.

It means a lot to fulfill my personal mission: "I help people experience enthusiasm, love and wisdom to fulfill Big Dreams."

When it comes to earning more while working less, consider being flexible and discover what you might do differently in a new stage in your life.

"You must be shapeless, formless, like water. When you pour water in a cup, it becomes the cup. When you pour water in a

bottle, it becomes the bottle. When you pour water in a teapot, it becomes the teapot. Water can drip and it can crash. Become like water, my friend." - Bruce Lee

3. Respect to inspect

My concept "respect to inspect" is about showing respect toward team members *by giving them what they need to succeed.*

I like the idea: "You can expect what you inspect." And I add to it: "Let your people know what you will be inspecting and what success will look like."

Tell them early as to what you *are* going to inspect.

In this way, you can follow the advice from Dr. Kenneth H. Blanchard: *"Help people reach their full potential. Catch Them Doing Something Right."*

When you lead a team, have you made sure that team members know what success looks like? Do they have the resources to make it happen?

4. Neutralize "occupational hobbies"

An "occupational hobby" is something you like to do that's related to your work but which is NOT your best task to do at this moment.

Some people like tinkering with Photoshop images when *it would be better for them to make phone calls to potential clients.*

So tinkering with Photoshop images is indulging in an occupational hobby instead of doing *the most productive, real work.*

What is your most productive, real work? What tasks are more like hobbies for you? Who can help you do the secondary tasks?

This section is about *Earn More and Work Less*. So delegating your "occupational hobbies" means that you

can focus on those tasks that help you earn more. And even better, you clear your calendar in many ways. You'll feel better and have more energy for your Drop-Weight Plan.

5. Make good budget decisions (face the pain)

Sometimes, to make the best budget decision, you have to make decisions that cause you some pain. For example, I made a decision that the budget for a *TimePulse* video was 3 hours for sound effects and mixing. If you view the video on YouTube and listen carefully, you'll discover that the bad guys who are kicked do NOT make a grunting sound like "Ugh!" Why? We ran out of time. Fortunately, the music and other sounds carry the day.

Still, it bothers me that an important ingredient was left out. But I've learned that it's necessary to make good decisions and prioritize details to guard a budget.

6. Open to new systems

To earn more and work less, it helps to implement an effective system. There are efficient ways to accomplish tasks and there are slower, clumsy ways. For example, many years ago, I worked in a bank. My co-worker only knew a particular spreadsheet program and he jumped to create a list in that program. However, it was much better to use a database program because this list would be used for many functions.

But my co-worker was *not* open to learning a new process/software to streamline about ten different needed outcomes.

To be open to systems is to stay aware and vigilant about finding ways to improve efficiency and accuracy.

7. Raise your fees

On the surface, the logic of raising your fees to earn more is practically inescapable. However, many of us hesitate to raise our fees because we're afraid that we'll lose our current clients.

The fear of losing clients when you raise your rates is often nothing more than an irrational fear. Every year that you're in business, you offer one more year of experience to your clients; one more year of learning; one more year of expertise. Doesn't that in itself justify at least an annual increase in your rates? Follow the advice above and your clients won't need to ask why, they'll simply know it's a standard part of your business policies. The one thing that most people say to me once they've broached the subject of raising their fees is this: "I can't believe I didn't do it sooner." I'm sure it will be the same for you. - Lea Woodward

Some years ago, when I first raised my coaching/consulting fee to $400, I was scared. The dialogue went like this:

Amanda: What's your fee?

Tom: (pushing himself past any hesitation) My place in the marketplace is $400 per hour.

Amanda: But the last person who worked on a speech with me was $75.00 per hour.

Tom: I hear you. And that's understandable. As I mentioned, my place in the marketplace is $400 per hour. Before our session, I'll send you questions that you'll answer so our time together will be especially valuable. We'll audio record your session because you won't have time to take notes. There will be *so much* information.

And I'll send you the recording, the MP3 file, through email. You can listen to our session again and again. And you'll get more and more value."

The above was a portion of the discussion. I soon guided the person to prepay for the session via credit card.

I've boiled down the process of raising your fees into a three-step process that I call "A.I.M. ":

Arrange rehearsal. Before the discussion of my fee, I rehearsed my phrase "My place in the marketplace is $400 per hour." The idea was for me to get over my fear and hesitation. I avoided any message of uncertainty. Clients want to know that *you know* your material and that you are good at what you do. They want to hear real confidence in your voice.

Intensify value. As you saw in the above dialogue, I mentioned my process that increases the value of the session. Providing the client with a recording of the session makes it possible for her to study the material again and again.

Measure your value. For my coaching, I have identified four areas:

G – get to the heart of it

A – acquire new knowledge

I – intensify systems

N – nurture new results

One reason to separate the coaching elements this way is because some coaching does not yield the full benefit until a month or more later. For example, when I help a client put in a new sales system, it may take a month before a significant increase in sales occurs.

Still, we can measure that the client acquired new knowledge (for example).

We can even measure details related to "intensify systems."

Questions can include:
- "On a scale of 1 to 5, did you have well-planned process for contacting and interacting with prospective clients?"
- "On a scale of 1 to 5, did you have a process for responding to a prospective clients' objections or tough questions?"

You need to give yourself evidence that what you do is truly worth the higher fee.

Furthermore, before you raise your fee, gather your testimonials. Use written and video-recorded testimonials to a great extent. Also, tell stories like: "Yes, I know I can help. For example, I had a client, Sarah, who had a similar tough situation . . ." Tell the rest of the story and demonstrate how you truly help people get powerful, positive results.

8. Empower hiring and delegating

"I only hire people who make my life easier," I said to a friend who asked me about how it feels to hire people.

I've learned to become skillful in "testing" people before I hire them. Here are three of a number of my methods:

a) I talk with the references and I ask questions like: "How did it go when something went wrong or was bumpy as you were working with Joe?" and "How did Joe do something to make things better?"

b) I give the person deadlines for getting back in touch with me. I observe carefully if they are trustworthy.

c) I listen carefully and I pay attention to my intuition.

Someone could be amazing at what they do, but if you don't like them, why bother hiring them? - Chip Conley

I have had to fire a couple of friends and so I'm truly careful about hiring people.

You have to be responsible when you're running an organization, and firing people who are your friends is part of that responsibility. - Ben Horowitz

Realize that if you hire well, you won't have to fire someone. For example, one of my friends wanted to work with me. This person had not been on time for any gathering of friends in seven years. I did *not* hire this friend, and she drifted away. I was sad to see her go, but I was glad that I had protected my work-life from the chaos her habits would have inflicted on my work-team. One detail that helped me make a good decision is my phrase: "I only hire people who make my life easier."

I didn't see it then, but it turned out that getting fired from Apple was the best thing that could have ever happened to me. The heaviness of being successful was replaced by the lightness of being a beginner again, less sure about everything. It freed me to enter one of the most creative periods of my life. - Steve Jobs

If you find that you have to fire someone, remember Steve Jobs' above comment that you may be helping the person transition into a better chapter of their life.

So it helps when you study methods about hiring, firing and delegating. Delegating is so important that we'll cover a whole section later in this book.

Here I'll emphasize that effective delegating requires *you to invest effort in training the person well* so you are freed from getting tangled in someone flailing about.

* * * * * *

We now turn to this next article because it concisely expresses some of the Earn More, Work Less concepts and strategies.

Law of Attraction and Earn More While You Work Less

Want to earn more? Learn to ask Empowering Questions.

The opposite is the Draining Question like: "Why does this always happen to me?"

Instead, ask an Empowering Question like: "How can I use this to make me stronger and smarter?"

Still, we can go to a higher level of asking questions. This higher level relates to asking questions connected to *3 Levels of Goals*.

3 Levels of Goals
- Good
- Excellent
- Outrageous-Good

Some of us say, "I'm realistic. If I sold 10 ebooks last month, I can aim for 15 ebooks this month." See the problem? A gain of 5 books does not feel exciting. How about an *Outrageous-Good* goal of 1,000 ebooks sold next month? How does that feel?

For many people, that would feel exciting! In fact, it was fun just to write "1,000 ebooks sold."

The point is: *Thinking of an Outrageous-Good goal leads to Empowering Questions.*

For example, one author set these goals: a) Good goal of 30 books sold, b) Excellent goal of 100 books sold, and c) Outrageous-Good goal of 3,000 books sold in one month.

This leads to the Empowering Question of *how could I possibly sell 3,000 books in one month?*

Such a question leads to a realization: *I need help.* Then, the author asks, "How can I get other authors to cross-promote with me so that we have several elists of subscribers alerted to the debut of my new book?"

Here's the pattern: 10 authors (with 5,000 esubscribers) leads to 50,000 people contacted and the potential for selling 1,000 books.

That's a good start.

Now it's your turn.

What might be an Outrageous-Good goal for you?

The Power of the Question "How can I pick projects with 'no ceiling' to value and prosperity?"

A few days ago, I had a haircut by a true artist. He took his time. Some hair stylists actually hit you in the head with the comb as they cut your hair. Not this gentleman. His hands were gentle, and the experience was calming.

Later, I had a sobering thought: No matter how well he does his job, this artist-hair stylist can only provide a limited number of haircuts per day. His prosperity hits a real limit.

Along this line, I guide my clients with this idea: *Some people get paid by the hour and others get "paid by leadership."* By this I mean, if you lead a team of people, you can make something—perhaps, a video or a book or even a song that can sell many copies. There is no ceiling.

But when you work by the hour, there is a ceiling to how much you can be paid.

For example, an attorney I know charges $425 per hour. However, another attorney charges $1500 for a kit to help business owners protect their assets. This attorney gives a speech to 2,000 people and 25% buy the kit. That's 500 purchases x $1500 which equals $750,000 in one hour. That is *no ceiling*.

Here are two more powerful questions to help you earn more while working less.

1) How can I find a topic that I *want* to study everyday?

To earn more, you need to become more valuable to the marketplace. How do you do that? You study a lot and learn more than most people on a specific topic.

This reminds me of a moment from the classic *Star Trek* 1960s television show: Captain Kirk found that he had to punish his chief engineer Scotty for getting into a brawl on a space station. Captain Kirk said, "Scotty, you're restricted to quarters until further notice."

Scotty replied, "Thank you, sir. That'll give me a chance to catch up on my technical journals!"

The point here is that Scotty *loved* studying technical details and he was the best in the galaxy as a chief engineer.

What do you want to excel at? (Earning more comes from being great at your profession.)

2) How can I find the intersection of what I'm Good At, what people Pay For, and Clients I Want?

Here's where the Law of Attraction really comes into play. The Law of Attraction holds that you attract what you think about most.

I've talked with clients who spend a lot of time complaining about their terrible customers (customers who cancel appointments and do not value their service). That's attracting the wrong clients!

This led me to form this Empowering Question: *How can I*

find the intersection of what I'm Good At, people Pay For, and **Clients I want?**

Now it's your turn.

Write in your journal the answer to the above question. Your answer may take the form of notes and even further questions.

Some of us do not work with clients directly. However, we work with people so you can adapt the question to "How can I work with people I prefer and earn more while working less?"

The Empowering Questions I've shared above turn the direction of our thoughts and help us, through the Law of Attraction, to attract the positive outcomes we want deep in our hearts.

Principle:

Use the Empowering Question: *How can I find the intersection of what I'm Good At, what people Pay For, and* **Clients I want?**

Power Question:

What would make it a joy to work with people? What are your best experiences with working with people? What are the characteristics of your best clients?

Now here are some guest articles about earning more:

The reason I'm sharing this article by Jeanna Gabellini is: Your ability to earn more begins with your habitual thinking patterns.

Billionaire Mentality
by Jeanna Gabellini

Do you want to increase your wealth and improve your relationship with money? Are you willing to ALLOW a constant flow of prosperity into your life?

All it takes is a decision and belief. Simple, huh?!

Sure, you'll have to let go of a great many negative beliefs that you currently hold on to for dear life.

Billionaires trust something that most people don't... there will always be an abundance of money and resources. A never-ending supply. They believe that all of their needs will be met. That includes money, love, knowledge, space, energy, peace, fun and more.

All billionaires may not feel all of that. But that is true prosperity. That "knowing and trust" allow you to act more freely. You make decisions based on what you want, not what is possible. Billionaires know it's all possible.

At any point so far have you thought ..

- I don't need to be a billionaire.
- I can't imagine that. A millionaire is even beyond me!
- How would I get there?
- That sounds overwhelming.

Prosperity means trusting that you can have the desired outcome without having to give up anything (except that nasty gremlin who has you believing those limiting thoughts!). When abundance is your primary belief, you can have it all. You won't be taking anything away from anyone else, either.

Recently, I went to a beautiful restaurant for dinner. The couple I was with kept making comments about the menu prices. It detracted from the beauty of the moment and anticipation of the meal. When you focus on price, you begin judging and justifying its worth.

If you're in business for yourself, you'll notice the same thing happens when you decide to increase your fee or your price list. If an expensive dinner freaks you out, don't do it. But notice what beliefs are making that decision for you. If you're focused on paying debt and cutting down on unnecessary expenses, this decision is aligned with your strategy. But strategy will only get you so far if you have lack lurking behind the scenes.

I've coached billionaires and millionaires, with no debt, and some are still plagued with the fear that someday their wealth will disappear. This has them making choices in their lives that aren't truly making them happy. They stay in careers where they work 24/7.

This is not the way life is designed to be. You have the choice to go on the same way or uncover more of what's limiting you. As you get smarter, the lack mentality is very subtle but has a huge impact on your life. The 'Billionaire Mentality' is available to you right now!

Are You Truly Ready For Prosperity? Really? You'll have bouts with fear, discomfort, and insecurity. You'll control, push, worry and get spun up in your head about how to get what you want.

It takes practice, but it's a worthy cause. And it can be quite fun!

Here are some small steps to get you started...

- Decide to focus on what you want, rather than on what you don't have.
- Ask yourself when making decisions, "If money wasn't an issue what would I do or how would I feel about this issue? If I knew my desire was possible what would I do next?"
- Surround yourself with people, books, audios and information that support you in this quest. This isn't the average person's way of thinking. Most people are hooked into struggle, limitation and "someday".
- Start noticing who is making decisions for you. Is it your "gremlin" or is it the "billionaire" in you who trusts in your brilliance and unlimited resources?

Jeanna Gabellini is a Master Business Coach who supports conscious entrepreneurs to double (and even triple) their profits by leveraging attraction principles, proven strategies and fun. She is also the co-author of *Life Lessons for Mastering the Law of Attraction*, with Eva Gregory, Mark Victor Hansen & Jack Canfield. And her newest book: *10 Minute Money Makers: How to Easily Double Your Profits in Just 10 Minutes a Day!*

Combining vision, divine guidance and easy to implement actions, Jeanna delivers top-tier private coaching & sold-out seminars that have allowed committed entrepreneurs to blow past their self-imposed limits, ditch the drama of overwhelm and move into radical joy, inner peace and ever-increasing profits.

Reach Jeanna through www.MasterPEACEcoaching.com

We learned about have the mental patterns to create great abundance in your life. Working with such inspiration from the above article, I'll now provide you a *principle* and *power question.*

Principle:
Focus on having trust that there is always money and abundance available.

Power Questions:
How can you shift your habitual thinking patterns to a "billionaire mindset" that focuses on positive possibilities to create more abundance? What reflexive negative thoughts do you want to drop? How will you capitalize on your inner brilliance?

* * * * * *

The reason I'm sharing this next article by C.J. Hayden is: To earn more, we need clarity and focused, positive actions.

Entrepreneur on a Mission?
Get Clear About What It Is
by C.J. Hayden

Congratulations! You've discovered you're an entrepreneur on a mission. But when someone asks you to explain what your mission is, it no longer seems as clear as it did when the light bulb first went on in your head. One's mission can be a slippery thing, morphing from one shape to another depending on the circumstance, and often seeming to defy words.

But if you can't define your mission clearly, you stand the risk of others defining it for you. Ideally, your entrepreneurial mission should help you determine what you want to accomplish. So when your mission remains foggy, your actions aren't always on target.

A clear mission helps you make decisions about what you do and don't want to do much more quickly. It acts like a lighthouse beacon, guiding you to find the navigable channel and avoid the rocks. This leads to higher productivity, better satisfaction, less frustration, and ultimately, making more of an impact.

A powerful entrepreneurial mission typically has three components:

1. Who you want to serve.
2. What you want for them as a result.
3. The wider impact or higher purpose of your actions.

Here are examples of clear missions from some of my coaching clients:

- Advise corporate executives on how to make their companies more socially responsible, increasing corporate social contribution worldwide.
- Help people with life-threatening illnesses get the medical care they deserve, transforming a broken health care system into one that works.
- Guide teenagers to develop their leadership skills so they can build stronger communities.
- Advise corporate executives on how to make their companies more socially responsible, increasing corporate social contribution worldwide.

And here are some examples, also from my coaching clients, of entrepreneurial missions that needed improvement:

- Advise small communities on how to keep their downtowns vital. (Who exactly is being served here? If you're not sure, you may not know who will hire you.)
- Train high-school students and teachers about sexual harassment. (What do you want for them as a result? When you can't express this, it's hard to sell it to anyone.)
- Sell energy conservation devices to conscious consumers online. (What's your purpose for doing this? Do you just want to make passive income or are you trying to make a social impact? When you aren't clear on this, it's hard to make strategic decisions or attract partners and supporters.)

When your mission is clearly defined, it shines its light on everything you do. It allows you to set worthwhile goals, design effective plans, evaluate new opportunities, and determine what's the most important thing to accomplish today.

Here are some coaching questions to ask yourself to get a clearer picture of your mission:

- Who do you truly want to serve? Whose goals and problems do you care about? Who do you enjoy reading about, hearing from, or spending time with? When you feel your blood boiling, whose situation has made you angry? Who do you feel deeply connected to, even when you don't know them?

- What result do you want to produce for those people? What do they need, want, and value? What unique contribution can you make to their situation? How can your gifts best be put to work?

- What is the wider impact or higher purpose of this work? Why do you want to do it? Why does it need to be done? How will the world be a better place if more of this work is in it? What legacy do you want to create for your life?

C.J. Hayden, MCC, CPCC, is the bestselling author of *Get Clients Now!, The One-Person Marketing Plan Workbook,* and over 400 articles. C.J. is a business coach and teacher who helps entrepreneurs get clients, get strategic, and get things done. Her company, Wings for Business, specializes in serving self-employed professionals and solopreneurs.

A popular speaker and workshop leader, C.J. has presented hundreds of programs on marketing and entrepreneurship to corporate clients, professional associations, and small businesses. She has taught marketing for John F. Kennedy University, Mills College, the U.S. Small Business Administration, and SCORE. She contributes regularly to dozens of magazines and websites, including Home Business, RainToday, and About.com.

We learned about getting real clarity about your mission in your business activities in the above article. Working with such inspiration, I'll now provide you with a *principle* and *power question.*

Principle:

To get a clearer picture of your mission, ask yourself questions related to whom you want to serve, what results you want to produce and what is your higher purpose.

Power Questions:

Do you know what your real mission is? Have you thought through not only whom you want to serve but what results you want to co-create with those clients?

* * * * * *

The reason I'm sharing the next article by Lois Creamer is: For many of us, being locked into being paid by the hour severely limits our free time for friends, family and our personal health practices. Lois addresses options for speakers and still the patterns she shares can help a number of people get into a "develop multiple streams of income" mindset.

Additional Revenue Streams
by Lois Creamer

You know from earlier posts [at my blog http://bookmorebusiness.com/blog/] that I consider you to be much more than a speaker. I consider you to be in the intellectual property business. Meaning, we get paid when we deliver (in whatever way) what it is that we know. It's all about delivering your expertise.

Your first revenue stream is, of course, your speaking fee. It is the one where you make the most profit. But it shouldn't be your **only** revenue stream.

Products really add to the bottom line. Make a live recording of your speech. Sell it as a CD or MP3 file. People love this kind of product!

Write a book. Books are a great way to share your intellectual property. I suggest you approach writing a book much like the old saying, "How do you eat an elephant? One bite at a time!"

Write an article on a dozen main points that you cover in a program/speech. Good size for articles is about 600 words. Embellish the article by adding a few stories that illustrate the point you are making. Then let's call it a chapter! Repeat a dozen times and you have a book! My approach makes it really doable. That's the key. A decision that must be made now is to publish with a publishing house, or to self-publish. More on that in a future post.

If you have a book, you have an eBook. I also share that you can take a collection of blog posts, tips and articles and create an eBook in days! I'll bet you have more content already than you realize.

How about taking your program and creating a companion workbook to go along with it? Then you have a type of "learning system". Perhaps a self-led version of your program.

Perhaps you have a program that could lend itself well to a licensing arrangement. By this I mean that someone else would deliver your program for you. Typically in this type of arrangement, a percentage of the fee is paid back to you. There are all sorts of ways people set up this type of plan.

You should be recording your speeches on a digital recorder and selling them. If people like what you have to say, they will want "more of you". You'll only gain from having speeches on CD's and MP3 files. Every product creates more interest in what you do.

I sent out a tweet that said: blog post = article = speech = book = eBook = learning system = licensing agreement = ??? I'm trying to point out that there is great value in leveraging your intellectual property in these ways. It is not only lucrative, but creative as well.

So, now that you are in an intellectual property business how are you going to leverage that property? Go out and create a new revenue stream now!

Lois Creamer is both small business strategist and specialist! She speaks from experience! Her clients have adopted her philosophy of concept and outcome marketing and use of positioning statement to successfully grow their businesses and increase profits. Her common sense ideas and high-energy approach make her a perfect choice for small business owners and entrepreneurs who want to learn new strategies that can be implemented immediately. Lois is the author of *Working Smart, Not Hard* as well as several audio programs.

Reach her at http://www.bookmorebusiness.com/

We learned you can start with one item and build a number of subsequent products from it—in the above article. Working with such inspiration from the above article, I'll now provide a *principle* and *power question*.

Principle:

Start with one item (perhaps a speech) and branch out into more products.

Power Question:

What topic really is close to your heart? Do you want to speak on that? Would you next consider recording the speech, then perhaps writing a related article or ebook?

* * * * * *

I am sharing this next article by Pat Baldridge because it reminds us that *to earn more we need to provide extraordinary benefits* for our clients and customers.

Create a Competitive Advantage When Proposing Your Talk
by Pat Baldridge

In my role as a meeting planner, one of my speakers gave me the best advice. He said, "How many of us motivate the audience at the time of our presentation, but know the enthusiasm will wane along with the good intentions to apply what was learned?" His suggestion was to announce a 30-day follow-up plan which includes three conference calls (with our speakers) and 30 days of a Facebook group that only audience participants can join. The conference call allows the speaker to share what s/he didn't have time to present and the Facebook group is a vehicle to share success stories (as they relate to what they learned) and stay connected with other attendees.

These two simple items would be a great value added when booking presentations.

Pat Baldridge is the President of the Charlotte Christian Chamber. Prior to her current role, Baldridge was a professional speaker, and management and sales trainer. Her list of prestigious clients include; Ford Motor Company, Baltimore Federal Executive Board, Carolina Health Systems, Dow Jones & Company, Duke Energy, Notre Dame College, Household Bank, Siecor Corporation and Sinai Hospital. Before establishing her own company, Pat worked with Dale Carnegie Training, Sandler Selling Systems, and the Management Development Group. A prolific writer, Pat has been published in the *Washington Business Journal*, the *Charlotte Observer*, *Warfield's Business Record* and was a regular columnist for *The Business Journal of Charlotte*. Her Ways to Win radio vignettes aired on numerous radio stations and provided solid solutions for workplace challenges. Baldridge's niche is to help managers and sales people build rapport using the Neuro Linguistic Programming model. As a 'connector' her passion is to encourage, engage, and equip Christian business professionals. She and her husband Dave reside in Charlotte, North Carolina.

We learned about the value of offering extra value. Working with such inspiration, I'll now provide you with a *principle* and *power question*.

Principle:
Look for ways to offer extra value and secure more business.

Power Question:
How can you do something extra that offers unique value to customers?

* * * * * *

We've covered the first part of the *Earn More, Work Less Equation*.

In the next chapter, we discuss strategies *so you can work less*.

Strategies so You Can Work Less
(and Have More Time to Lose Weight)

As my sweetheart and I stepped out of her car, preparing to walk across the Golden Gate Bridge, I had an image pop into my mind. What if a huge hive stood like a mountain in the center of the Golden Gate Bridge? This image became the center of my collection of science fiction stories in my book *TimePulse: Beyond Titanic.*

I've learned that many of my best creative ideas arise after or *during* a period of time when I'm relaxing and refreshing my mind and body.

* * *

Have you noticed that some people just keep pouring on more work so they're always busy?

To put it simply, it takes real focus, strategy and discipline to *work less.*

When you work less, you can fill your time with health-enhancing activities like taking a walk with a loved one, enjoying a yoga class, or going for a refreshing bicycle ride.

We'll use the W.O.R.K.L.E.S.S. process

W – Work out your identity

O – organize training

R – revitalize work to be a joy (transform)

K – keep listening

L – let go

E – empower team members

S – select only what you do best (delegate)

S – set criteria for excellence and "set breaks to create breakthroughs"

1. Work out your identity

If you are your work, *then who are you when you're not working?* For so-called workaholics, this may be a big hurdle to get over. Why? Some of us only feel safe when we're really busy. That's when we feel like we're "good people."

To work less, means stretching the "I'm only good if I'm busy" story of yourself into a New Story.

Such a New Story is: *I have intrinsic goodness. I'm good when I'm working, playing, and just sitting and "being" in this moment.* What does "being" mean, anyway? It means to experience a spiritual side of yourself—that part of you which is connected with the goodness of the universe. It takes practice to slow down and be conscious of an inner peace.

An important note: When you work less and have more time, be careful to avoid falling into the trap of mind-numbing activities like watching a lot of television. Remember, your plan to work less and have more time is about doing *Life-enhancing* activities like taking a walk with a loved one. Be sure to exercise. Move, move, move!

2. Organize training

To work less, you need to delegate certain tasks to well-trained team members. It *does* take significant time and effort to make sure a team member is trained and equipped to succeed at doing a task. Still, providing good training is essential if you want more time to take care of yourself.

I've heard many people say, "I don't have time to train somebody else. I'd rather do it myself and just get it done."

This is a thought pattern that really limits a number of people's lives. To work less, have more time, and to ultimately get more done, we need to have well-trained people supporting us.

3. Revitalize work to be a joy (transform)

An interesting way to "work less" is to actually enjoy your work where much of it becomes "play." Earlier in this book, I wrote about a great question: *"How can you make your work about something you're Good At, people will Pay For, and with Clients You Want?"* The elements of "good at" and "clients you want" will enliven your positive feelings. Then work feels joyful and your productivity rises. More productivity gives you the opportunity to choose more time off.

Researchers have noted that many highly productive people actually work less hours. How can that be? Because a number of people work long hours even though a significant amount of that time is "grinding with no productivity." It's often better to go home, rest, and come in early the next day.

Now it's your turn.
Where is the joy in your work?

For example, I often write fast and well after I've seen an inspiring episode of one of my favorite TV shows. I'm full of inspiration and energy, and I then write quickly and clearly. So I start with joy and then I sit down and write.

4. Keep listening

Ineffective listening creates complication and a waste of time. How? Confusion arises when people do not listen well.

How can you do more listening? Ask good questions. When you want to work less, you ask questions like:
- "What do you need so you'll succeed with this project?"
- "What do you need me to know?"
- "Is the deadline realistic?"
- "I want you to succeed. Can you foresee a problem that you might have?"
- "What is working for you in this team?"
- "What do you feel might need an adjustment?"

Listen well. Then look for a way to say sincerely "I agree" to some detail. Saying "I agree" puts the other person at ease and builds your relationship with him or her. Why does "I agree" have such power? The reason is that many of us spend so much time trying to prove that we're right. When we hear someone say, "I agree" then we know we can stop with pushing our point of view.

5. Let go

Do you want to work less? Fire people who do not fit with what your team is doing.

Author Dan Kennedy suggests that the best time to fire a team member is the first time you're thinking about it. That may appear extreme, but Dan is pointing out that your team members should not be causing you to lose sleep. Team members need to be doing their jobs correctly and for the benefit of the team and customers.

Let go of the idea that because you feel scared or uncomfortable you cannot do an action. You may feel uncomfortable about "letting go" of a disruptive employee, but let them go. All of the successful people I have interviewed alerted me to the fact that they took action even when afraid or unsure.

Further, *let go* is the central idea of starting to work less. Let go of always trying to look good to others or gain their approval. Identify *who you really are* and what you really value. Happiness, success and time to take care of your body (lose weight) depend on you **letting go** of putting other things before your own health.

6. Empower team members

A prime way so that you personally work less is for you to empower other team members to get things done. For example, author Tim Ferris empowered his customer service representatives to solve problems in ways that could cost up to $100.00. If the representative could solve the problem by sending $100.00 worth of product to a disgruntled customer, then the representative could easily resolve the problem without Tim getting involved. This gave Tim Ferris more time to focus on other things important to him when it came to his work and his life

I always remember a line from the 1960's Classic *Star Trek* television show. Dr. McCoy tells Captain Jim Kirk: "Jim, let your people do their jobs."

7. Select only what you do best (delegate)

To work less, it helps for you to do, as much as possible, *only what you do the best*. You have natural talents that bring you up to, perhaps, the top 15% of people who do that particular activity. For example, many business owners are the best people to make sales presentations for their company. That means they do better by delegating the bookkeeping to a team member or a contractor. One top real estate agent only works four days a week while her two team members do the other work like pre-qualifying potential clients.

It takes effort and the ability to face reality, to identify what you do best and what, if you have a business, requires only you to take action. Make that effort and delegate other activities. (Delegating is so important that, later in this book, I share more insights about the process.)

8. Set criteria for excellence and "set breaks to create breakthroughs"

Setting criteria for excellence frees you from trying to "do things perfectly." This will save you a lot of time and help you work less. Again, we're focused on working less so we can do more to take care of our body.

We do not have time to do everything perfectly. Many things do not have to be perfect—for example, a draft of a report that you know the team will work on this afternoon.

(Yes, one can find an exception to the "it does not need to be perfect" idea. Surgery needs special attention. I'm grateful that a surgeon did excellent work that helped my mother recover the use of her hands and legs!)

To *Set Criteria for Excellence* ask yourself (or a team) these questions:

- What is most important for this project to succeed?
- What can we drop from this project?
- If we're doing triage (like battlefield medicine), what needs to be done first?

- What do the stakeholders (clients, supervisors) most care about? How can we fulfill their expectations?

Now we'll focus on "set breaks to create breakthroughs." With this phrase, I'm referring to the phenomenon that taking a break often refreshes our brain and body to be doubly creative and productive upon our return to work.

To help you work less, be strategic about taking a break. In college, I could study twelve hours a day for finals because I used a 50/10 rule. 50 minutes of studying then 10 minute break. I kept a log. Often, my break would be walking outside around the college library.

* * * * * *

Now here are guest articles about working less:

(Remember: when you work less, you have more time and energy for health-enhancing activities.)

The reason that I'm sharing the next article by C.J. Hayden is: To *work less*, we need to focus on doing the most effective actions and avoiding time-consuming mistakes.

From Conversation to Client in Four Simple Steps

by C.J. Hayden

Our lives as professionals marketing our own services would be much easier if clients would simply read our sales copy and decide to hire us. But in the real world, it rarely works that way. Instead, we must have conversations with our prospects before a sale takes place—sometimes several conversations.

These selling conversations can seem difficult or intimidating, but they don't have to be. Here are four simple steps to turn conversations into paying clients.

Step 1. What do you need?

Keys to success: Being curious. Listening. Letting go of assumptions.

Begin every sales conversation by asking prospects to tell you about their needs, and listen carefully to what they tell you. Forget about what you think they should want, and pay attention to what they really do want.

Common mistakes: Starting with Step 2 instead, or beginning Step 2 too soon.

Even when prospects start the conversation by asking you to describe your services, take a moment to find out more about them first. When prospects tell you their problems and goals, they are handing you the secrets of how to sell to them successfully.

Step 2. Here's what I have.

Keys to success: Matching what you have to what they need as specifically as possible.

Describe your services in direct response to the needs your prospects tell you about. If they're in a hurry, tell them how you can work quickly. If they want accuracy, describe your attention to detail. Use the same words and phrases they used, and speak to the same issues they did.

Common mistakes: Sharing features and processes instead of benefits and results.

When prospects ask how you work, what they really want to know is what results you produce, not the steps you follow to get there. They want to hear what benefits your services have for them, not an inventory of all the bells and whistles included in your service package.

Step 3. Is there a match?

Keys to success: Collaborating with your prospect. Consulting or coaching instead of persuading.

You'll make more sales when you and your prospects are on the same side, instead of being adversaries. Act as if they have already hired you, and help them solve their problem. Don't just talk about how you could help; show them what it's like to work with you.

Common mistakes: Ignoring your prospects' concerns. Becoming defensive. Trying to coax prospects to buy.

Every concern a prospect has is legitimate. Acknowledge each one and explore together what resolution might be possible. Stay focused on their needs instead of your own. Trying to convince prospects you know more about what's right for them than they do will backfire.

Step 4. Will you hire me?

Keys to success: Asking a yes or no question, then waiting for an answer.

Once you've completed the first three steps, it's time to ask your prospects if they are ready to work with you. Be sure you've resolved their concerns from Step 3. Ask a direct question; don't wait for them to offer. Then stop talking until they reply.

Common mistakes: Asking too soon. Not asking at all. Giving them reasons not to buy.

Don't talk yourself out of a sale by bringing up their concerns again when you ask if they're ready to get started. For example, "Would you like to work with me? I know you said the price was higher than you planned, but..." Just ask, and wait.

The good news is that once you arrive at Step 4, the answer is rarely "no." If your services aren't a good fit for your prospects' needs, you'll find that out by the time you get to Step 3. (And in that case, you won't be asking for their business at all.) You're more likely to hear a reason they wish to delay their decision. Help them determine a timeframe for making up their minds, and set a date to resume the conversation at Step 3.

If selling conversations are challenging for you, rehearse these steps with a friend, colleague, or coach playing the role of prospect. Once you become more comfortable with the process, you'll find your prospects begin to relax also, and these conversations will become easier for both of you. And that will lead naturally to more sales.

C.J. Hayden, MCC, CPCC, is the bestselling author of *Get Clients Now!, The One-Person Marketing Plan Workbook,* and over 400 articles. C.J. is a business coach and teacher who helps entrepreneurs get clients, get strategic, and get things done. Her company, Wings for Business, specializes in serving self-employed professionals and solopreneurs.

A popular speaker and workshop leader, C.J. has presented hundreds of programs on marketing and entrepreneurship to corporate clients, professional associations, and small businesses. She has taught marketing for John F. Kennedy University, Mills College, the U.S. Small Business Administration, and SCORE. She contributes regularly to dozens of magazines and websites, including Home Business, RainToday, and About.com.

We learned simple steps to getting clients faster and with leas effort. Working with such inspiration I'll now provide you with a *principle* and a *power question.*

Principle:
Develop a specific plan for your selling conversation and rehearse with a friend.

Power Question:
How can you simplify and clarify how you talk about your product or service?

* * * * * *

The reason I'm sharing this next article by Jeff Davidson is: To demonstrate how you can become credible to someone you may partner with (which will save you time). This particular article relates to speakers and speaker bureaus; however, I invite you *to observe the patterns in which you can create credibility.*

Attracting Speakers Bureaus
by Jeff Davidson

Gaining in-depth knowledge of the bureau business is an excellent prelude to being represented by bureaus. All other things being equal, why do some speakers attract the attention of bureaus more than others? Independent of your topic, experience, location, fee structure, or any other particulars of your situation, the components that follow will help make you more attractive to bureaus:

• Be requested by their clients. Nothing else compares to this component of attracting bureau business. When you make presentations and clients call bureaus asking them to book you, that in and of itself is the strongest indicator of your viability in the marketplace. When the same bureau gets multiple calls for your services, it conveys an indelible message. So, become as good as you can: practice, practice, practice. Speak to many groups and leave them amazed, inspired, and ready for more.

• Have tremendous video footage. Are you already a household name? Then you need no video, and you are attractive to bureaus. Otherwise, you need to video record yourself on many occasions, and extract the best of the best. While the video itself does not need to be more than 11 or 12 minutes, the segments must be compelling.

• Send them a client. Bureau owners and booking agents are appreciative of people with long memories. If you send them a client—a company that is ready to book a speaker for a particular engagement on a specific date—you have established the basis for a beautiful friendship with that bureau. Sending a regular stream of clients to the bureau increases your chances of becoming one of their favorite speakers.

• Simply diverting business their way will be for naught if you have not honed your speaking skills to a fine edge. Hereafter, whenever you get a call from a meeting planner, and you are not quite the right speaker for the engagement, turn over the lead to your favorite bureau. This is a triple-win situation with a potential long-term payoff.

• Have tremendous word-of-mouth. Meeting planners and bureaus discuss excellent speakers and hot topics. If no one has called a bureau specifically requesting your services, and you haven't sent any particular clients to a bureau, you might find that they are still highly interested in your speaking capabilities based on word-of-mouth recommendations. Bureau reps talk to one another, to people in the meeting planning industry, and to other speakers. If your name keeps coming up in a favorable light, it is to your benefit. The way to make this happen is to be so good on the podium that people simply start talking about you. That takes years of practice, refinement, coaching, and honing your craft, but you can do it.

• Be in the news. Diligent professional bureau representatives read their own industry trade magazines and articles. If a speaker is featured in such publications, bureaus could become interested in him or her. As speakers, we take pride in the long years that we spend on the road speaking to audiences and getting better at making presentations. Yet, the most-popular and highest-priced speakers often are those who have the benefit of being in the news.

• Have a monopoly on a topic. If you're the sole expert in the world on a topic that happens to be in vogue, then you have positioned yourself well. If you're one of a handful of experts on a particular topic, that can also work.

• Be recommended by their friends. Similar to having great word-of-mouth, being recommended by a friend of the bureau is a master stroke in your marketing campaign. Suppose that you do well for Bureau ABC, and you ask the owner or agent to put in a good word for you at Bureau DEF. If he or she obliges, you have tremendous inroad with Bureau DEF. People tend to value the recommendations of friends and people whom they trust.

• Get them to like you. This is harder than it sounds. All of human psychology tells us that people are more inclined to do business with people they like. If you're regarded as likeable, a true and sincere friend, someone who adds value and otherwise embodies all of the other aspects of what friendship entails, you increase your probability of doing business with any particular bureau.

Jeff Davidson, aka "The Work-life Balance Expert"® offers keynote presentations and workshops on a creating work-life balance, managing the pace with grace, and thriving in a hyper-accelerated world. Jeff is the author of *Simpler Living, Breathing Space,* and *Dial it Down, Live it Up.* visit www.BreathingSpace.com

We learned about doing the essentials so people want to team up with us—in the above article. Working with such inspiration, I'll now provide you with a *principle* and *power questions.*

Principle:

Find out how you can stand out and be trustworthy to the person you're contacting.

Power Questions:

What do you uniquely bring to the marketplace? How might you team up with other people once they know your unique skills and trustworthiness?

Delegate

(And Save Your Time
so You Have More Personal Energy
to Focus on Your Health-enhancing Activities)

Milly read a book on management and nodded her head many times while looking at the section on "delegating." But things were falling apart. She was afraid to fire two people because then she might look like she was a poor manager. So she "ran like crazy" trying to cover for mistakes of the two troublesome team members. She cut out her exercise classes and found herself awake late at night and turning to food.

Her inner peace was falling and her weight was climbing.

I've taken care with this section on delegating because I've personally learned that **work, pressure and upsets caused by trouble with team members can lead to overeating**. Delegate well and you have more positive energy. Delegate poorly and you are now in a "red alert" mode of living. I have seen business people get promotions and suddenly get fatter and fatter. Leading people, without using good strategies, can be extremely stressful. As a result,

175

a number of managers cut out their exercise-time, trying to cover for mistakes done by people who report to them.

When you delegate well, *work gets done, but you're not physically there.*

On occasion I watch a TV show *Restaurant Impossible.* I have no intention to own a restaurant at this time. (I do not say a definitive "no.") My hesitation about having a restaurant is the problem that employees don't always show up. Then an owner must go in and cover for any employee who fails to work their shift. This just adds more work to the owner's plate.

Instead, I prefer moments when I have three illustrators working on different parts of a graphic novel and four colorists work on other sections. Simultaneously, I have two editors working on my next non-fiction book. And at this moment, I have a video editor editing my DVD *The 3 C's of Success: Charisma, Confidence and Control of Time.*

All of those team members can be working, while I'm exercising, sleeping or perhaps, in a classroom teaching college students.

When I delegate well, I can do something I love to do in San Francisco—visit with friends.

I delegate every day. And I've delegated elements of projects since the first short film I made at nine years old.

We'll use the D.E.L.E.G.A.T.E. process:

D – decide what you will NOT do
E – engage training
L – listen
E – expect and inspect
G – give a Clear Measurement
A – act as you want them to act
T – "test" before you hire

E – express and confirm deadlines and "criteria for excellence"

1. Decide what you will NOT do

An important process is to "eliminate occupational hobbies." An occupational hobby is something you like to do but it's something that does not represent your best talent nor the best use of your time. For example, one of my clients, Moira likes working with Photoshop. However, she has a team member Sam who could do her html-enewsletter with images better and faster than she could. As the leader of her company, her time is better focused on getting more clients.

People talk of focusing on priorities. I'm also interested in identifying "droppables." We do not have time for everything so we must be selective.

Here are some things that you might aim to drop:
- bookkeeping
- routine household maintenance items
- mowing the lawn

Now it's your turn.

What are the tough things that you need to focus on? What routine tasks should you delegate?

2. Engage training

Measure twice cut once. – English Proverb

I refer to this classic proverb because training done well is like being careful and measuring twice. If you measure wrong, you could waste some expensive lumber.

If you do a slip-shod effort at training someone, you could waste a lot of time trying to minimize the damage caused by a poorly trained team member.

You start reaping time-savings *after* you've sown the

seeds for excellent performance. How? You sow the seed of excellent training *and* verify that the person truly knows how to do the process effectively and create the good results you seek.

On the other hand, many people do *not* train the team member thoroughly and do *not* verify that the person really understands what he or she is doing. The result is: confusion and wasted time.

Do *not* let that happen. Instead, make sure to ask questions. Have the person show you how they really understand the training and that they're ready to do a great job. I say, "Let me see if I was clear in what I shared with you. When you get to Step 2 you will . . .?" I double check that the person can do the tasks well.

3. Listen

To listen well, it helps to ask effective questions. I often ask a team member, "Is there anything else I need to know?"

I also ask, "Is there anything you need from me so you can succeed?"

In my keynote addresses, I point out **Three Listening Blockers.**

Listening Blocker #1: Defending. People naturally push back. They try to protect themselves. Unfortunately, in that moment, they are not listening.

Listening Blocker #2: Judging. Researchers define the brain stem as the "reptile brain." Its focus is on survival. So we naturally scan every word, gesture and facial expression to see if someone may hurt us. We're judging all of the time. The problem is that such judgments can put a wall between us and other people. And those others can see the judgmental thoughts as disturbing facial expressions and vocal tones.

Listening Blocker #3: Me too, One Up. Many of us have heard adults say things like: "Oh. I understand how tough it is to have a newborn baby. I have newborn twins." That's "one up." Even worse, that's taking over the "spotlight" of the conversation.

The solution is to pause and take a breath. Then ask a question. Turn the "spotlight" of the conversation back onto the other person.

The excellent manager makes sure to listen because listening shows respect and appreciation for a team member.

How does the person know that you heard him or her? You use what I call a *Reflective Reply.* That's when you say something like:

- That sounds intense. How did you feel about that?
- That sounds frustrating.

Some people suggest that emotions are to be kept out of the workplace. On the other hand, numerous researchers and authors show how people really are emotional even if they attempt to hide it in the workplace.

An old phrase is: *People buy on emotions and later justify on fact.*

The same happens with your team members. If you listen to them, they are more likely to "buy in" to your direction and leadership.

To my audiences, I emphasize: *When you're listening, you're winning.*

"Everyone has an invisible sign hanging from their neck saying, 'Make me feel important.' Never forget this message when working with people. - Mary Kay Ash

4. Expect and inspect

You can expect what you inspect. When you delegate, the process is ***not*** "set and forget." No! The process is train well and set up "natural check-in points." When I work with contractors and interns, we're always setting deadlines. A few minutes ago, I was talking with one of my illustrators. He is working on a complicated action sequence for the big ending of one of the graphic novels of the *Jack AngelSword* series I created. I told him, "We'll talk tomorrow. Don't worry. Tell me when you get stuck. I can provide you with a bridge or at least a band-aid to make the pieces come together."

I prefer to *avoid* hovering: I set it up that contractors can send me an email when they have a particular section of a project done. I do not hover, but I'm sure to set a good deadline with person. Before we're done setting the deadline, I ask, "Is this realistic? Is there some way that you can see a problem coming up?"

All of the contractors reporting to me know that I will inspect their work.

I once had a particular accountant work for me. I double-checked his work and found a $400.00 error. My team members know that I double-check the work.

I tell my illustrators, "Our team members are watching each other's back. We want you to do work that you're proud of."

Remember: You can expect what you inspect.

5. Give a Clear Measurement

People perform better when they know exactly what is required. Clear measurements can include:
- 30 days with zero accidents
- 10 marketing phone calls per day

- Find ways to earn an average of $250 per day (or X-amount per week)

Now it's your turn.

How can you provide a simple measurement so that you and the team know if you're succeeding or not?

6. Act as you want them to act

Be on time and people will be on time. Respond quickly to email and many times team members will reciprocate. But show sloppiness and you'll get that bad outcome from other people.

Hold yourself to high standards and you show team members how you operate in your company.

7. "Test" before you hire

I pay close attention to the behavior of a potential intern or contractor before I hire him or her.

My "tests" are about whether the person's actions align with my principle: "I only hire people who make my life easier." Another way to say this: "I do *not* hire people who are *not* trustworthy to act in a reliable way."

One of the tests is: I give potential interns a series of deadlines for staying in contact with me. I observe whether the internship candidate is conscientious in meeting those deadlines.

In years of hiring and paying interns, I have only had four interns not work out. Not a bad average. But those four situations left a mark on me. So I now provide a statement, *"Supplemental Information for an Internship"*

Some of the provisions in the Supplemental Information include:

"2. With each internship customized toward helping the

intern's career, the internship depends on how the intern participates in making the internship extremely valuable.

To say this in few words, like many things in life, what you get out of it depends on what you put into it.

3. There is a lot of flexibility in the schedule in that the intern can specify that he or she needs to step away for a week or two related to midterm exams and final exams and other important life events.

4. According to the research, a job applicant with "internship" on the resume has a 17% advantage.

5. Since this is an internship, certainly interns must do some work that specifically relates to deadlines and priorities of Tom Marcoux Media, LLC. Some of these duties may be routine or not "fun."

6. One of the goals is for the intern to do work that is very useful for the intern's portfolio.

7. Tom Marcoux feels that he takes on a personal commitment to each intern who is hired for an internship.

8. To "quit the internship" before a successful completion of the 150 hours is a serious decision and can be considered "breaking one's word." So potential interns are advised to carefully make their decision about whether they submit their application to the internship. It is better to say "no" to the internship opportunity than to go into the internship with a "half-commitment."

9. During the internship, we use a process that reduces stress and pressure—Expected Completion Date (ECD). When we talk about a subproject—together we come up with a reasonable estimate of when the subproject (like two quick thumbnail sketches) will be completed.

You will be in discussion with Tom Marcoux and you can say something like: 'Oh, I have family visiting so I expect that I can complete it by Wednesday Oct. 16th, 10 pm.'"

Another situation that is similar to "hiring" someone is to decide whether to team up with another small business owner. Test whether such a team up is a good idea by doing a small "pilot project." It is important to get past wishful thinking about teaming up with another person.

Sometimes, I make this analogy: "Do not marry someone without going on an extended vacation with them first. Discover two things: Are they flexible? Are they kind?"

By doing a small pilot project, you give yourself a chance to see how the other person responds or reacts to pressure.

It's better to make an informed decision.

Special Note: **Hiring the wrong person or teaming up with another small business owner who causes you trouble may lead you to lose lots of time and sleep . . . and it may even create stress that makes you vulnerable to overeating.**

I'm being quite specific in this section so that you can work less and devote more time to health-enhancing activities.

8. Express and confirm deadlines and "criteria for excellence"

If you don't confirm deadlines, then you have nothing to hold the team member to. It gets worse. People do *not* like uncertainty. They actually feel better when they know boundaries and requirements of the job.

"Everyone needs deadlines. Even the beavers. They loaf around all summer, but when they are faced with the winter deadline, they work like fury. If we didn't have deadlines, we'd stagnate."
– Walt Disney

Years ago, I felt uncomfortable and hesitated in naming deadlines. Then I learned that I could make it a winning experience for the team member. I have said, "Let's set the deadline. We'll make it realistic. If you complete the section early, you'll be a hero. I want you to succeed."

Dr. Ken Blanchard says, "Catch people doing something right." I add, "When you set good deadlines with the person's input, you make it possible for the person do something right."

When I speak of *Criteria for Excellence*, I'm talking about focusing on the most important elements of the project. We simply do not have time for everything. So we need to target what is most important to people affected by the project. What is most important to the client? To the supervisor? To yourself and your team members?

Some people suggest what is most important is: "Protect the job." Also, people include: "do the ethical thing!"

Still, what can you drop from the project? I call these "droppables." Be sure you check in with the "stakeholders" (supervisor, client, etc.) *before* you drop something because that element may be close to their heart.

When you delegate, make sure you clearly communicate what is most important to you for the project. Ask your team member, "So I know that I was clear: What is the Criteria for Excellence for this project?" Listen to the team member's response. It is often surprising, even alarming, how other people misinterpret what we say.

Be sure to go a "couple of rounds" in your discussion so that you're sure the person understands the Criteria for Excellence. *Devoting time at the beginning* of the project saves you from unnecessary trouble at the end of the project.

Devote effort around Criteria for Excellence.

Special Note: Using Criteria for Excellence is a powerful way to guard your time so that you make sure to exercise daily.

Now here are guest articles related to delegating and better communication:

Some of us need to develop better communication skills and habits so that we can delegate more effectively. Sometimes, a team member makes a serious mistake and it's hard not to react with harsh words. That's why I'm sharing this following article by Rebecca Morgan.

Is Your Communication Strategic?
by Rebecca Morgan, CSP, CMC

In a recent "Calming Upset Customers" seminar, I explained why people go ballistic when angry.

"When we're upset, we behave from our emotions and have cut off all rational thinking. A rational person would think, 'How can I best accomplish my communication goal?' It would not be by yelling or cursing at the person who can possibly find a solution."

Afterward, the participants' discussion made me realize that few people think about a communication strategy before they open their mouths. Most people just spew forth whatever crosses their mind, with little or no thinking or filter — especially when upset.

How can you not fall prey to this predisposition? How can you be more cognizant of your communication goal so you don't get caught in emotional triggers?

1. Before entering what you think may become a contentious situation, take a moment to remind yourself what you want to accomplish. Ask yourself, "What is the best strategy for accomplishing my communication goal?"

2. If you have any history of raising your voice, cursing, or becoming argumentative, ask yourself, "How can I not get triggered and become emotional?" Perhaps you need to remind yourself to breathe, pause before responding, ask questions before reacting, and ask for the other person's help.

3. If you find yourself getting angry say something like, "I'm getting frustrated. I'd like to escalate this to your manager before this conversation gets heated." Or if with a coworker, "I can feel myself getting tense which diminishes rational thinking. I'd like to take a few minutes to collect my thoughts and then resume this discussion."

By thinking through your communication goals and creating a strategy, you are more likely to have a satisfying interaction. Even if you don't get what you want, you know you've behaved maturely and haven't embarrassed yourself nor unthinkingly berated someone else.

Rebecca L. Morgan, CSP, CMC, specializes in creating innovative solutions for customer service challenges. She's appeared on *60 Minutes, Oprah, the Wall Street Journal, National Public Radio* and *USA Today*. Rebecca is the bestselling author of 25 books, including *Calming Upset Customers* and *Professional Selling*. She is an exemplary resource who partners with you to accomplish high ROI on your strategic customer service projects. For information on her services, books, and resources, or for permission to repost or reprint this article, contact her at 408/998-7977, Rebecca@RebeccaMorgan.com,
http://www.RebeccaMorgan.com/

We learned about preplanning our communication and focusing on "how can I not be triggered and become emotional?"—in the above article. Working with such inspiration, I'll now provide you with a *principle* and *power question*.

Principle:
Excellent communication requires preplanning and strategy.

Power Question:
What do you need to think through *before* you communicate with someone?

* * * * * *

The reason I'm sharing this article by Craig Harrison is: To communicate well and build good work relationships, it's essential to praise well.

Be A Praise Dispenser:
Employ the Power of Praise
To Reward and Incent
By Craig Harrison

Workplace surveys constantly remind us that what employees realistically want more than money, titles and corner offices, is recognition and appreciation. They want to be noticed. They want to be appreciated. They want recognition for their efforts. So simple, yet so wanting.

What does it cost to praise an employee, recognize a colleague or acknowledge appreciation of someone else's efforts? According to Cindy Ventrice, author of *Make Their Day! Employee Recognition That Works:* "57 percent of the most meaningful recognition received is absolutely free. No budget, special equipment or legislation is required. Just a willingness to extend oneself." Toastmasters around the world already understand this.

Many coaching clients confide in me their manager doesn't recognize them or their relationship partner isn't praiseworthy, and thus they feel unappreciated. Yet when I ask them if they praise their own direct reports, or compliment their mate, they sheepishly reply: "On occasion." Other times they murmur: "That's not my style" or simply say "They know I appreciate them." Herein lies the problem.

Some of us grew up in environments devoid of positive feedback. We've come to believe we either don't deserve it, or perhaps convince ourselves we don't need it. We tell ourselves: "I'm tough, I'm strong." After all, we're adults. We're professionals! We don't need the strokes or handholding. Payment is our reward. Yet our ability to receive praise when given feeds our foundation of success.

The Power of Praise

A heartfelt compliment, genuine kudos or a well-placed pat on the back goes a long way toward expressing the appreciation you feel. American humorist, writer and playwright Mark Twain stated it well: "I can live for two months on a good compliment."

There's power in the praise you give to those in your life. And a funny thing happens, too. When you give it to others you get it back in return. Whether recognition comes from the party you praised, or elsewhere, payback is a beautiful thing!

Praise The Toastmaster

Toastmasters understand the power of praise more than most. In our evaluations we temper our criticism with praise for what a speaker is already doing effectively. We sandwich criticism with praise on either side to ensure recipients internalize that which they've done well. (I've heard it jokingly called "kiss 'em, kick 'em and kiss 'em.")

Payment in Praise

Let's face it, in Toastmasters we don't have lavish budgets to dispense bonuses for members doing things right or performing roles well. We can't give members promotions to new offices, extra vacation time or fanciful titles as rewards for commendable performance. But we can certainly lavish them with well-deserved praise, both publicly and privately. It's a powerful form of currency we as humans are under-utilizing.

According to Dr. Elayne Savage, Psychotherapist, communication coach and author of *Don't Take It Personally* —*The Art of Dealing with Rejection:* "Praise is both a reward and a motivation. If we don't get rewarded for certain behavior we'll start slacking off. We don't try quite as hard or put as much energy or time into it. We all want the attention. The bottom line: we need that validation, whether we admit it or not. We need the reward."

Dr. Savage, a member of Emeryville Toastmasters continues: "Praise is also a motivator to do more things, think out of the box, be creative, or whatever we've been complimented on. We enhance those qualities. That's why it's important to be specific when giving praise. Specific praise given will inform the direction a person grows in. They receive it and decide Oh, this is what's important!"

Not All Praise Is Equal!

The power of praise derives from the combination of words spoken and their source. When your buddy says "good job" it may not carry the same cache as a similar acknowledgement from your club president or area governor. In the work world recognition from managers (from supervisor to senior management) accounts for a full 70 percent of the most meaningful recognition employees receive, according to Cindy Ventrice, workplace recognition expert and author of *Make Their Day*.

So be advised: your words of support for other Toastmasters carry the weight of what you say, how you say it, who else hears it and who you, the issuer of the praise, is. If you, as a veteran Toastmaster, praise a newcomer it will simultaneously encourage and inspire them.

PEZ: Praise & Encourage with Zeal

Ultimately, we as Toastmasters, like those popular Pez candy dispensers, can reward achievement with praise and also leave a sweet taste in achievers' mouths that leaves them poised to earn more!

Putting the Power of Praise into Action: Steps to Success

Identify colleagues, co-workers and others who are praiseworthy.

Now deliver heartfelt praise, whether privately or publicly.

Don't combine praise with criticism—it diminishes or even negates the praise.

Beware of hyperbole. Simply give your praise honestly and with love.

("He who praises everybody, praises nobody." — Samuel Johnson)

See the reaction of the person you are praising.

Meanwhile, how do you feel when you have praised someone else?

Congratulations, you've just become a Praise Dispenser and created a win-win.

Praise be thou!!!

Craig Harrison's ExpressionsOfExcellence.com provides sales and service solutions for organizations and communication and leadership development for individuals. Based in the San Francisco Bay Area, Craig is a speaker, trainer, author, consultant, coach and storyteller and an active leader in the National Speakers Association, Toastmasters International and National Storytelling Network

* Download Craig's free Quick Start Guide to finding the best Toastmasters club for you!

www.ExpressionsOfExcellence.com/Toastmasters/QuickStartGuide_Toastmasters.pdf

We learned about the value and mechanics of praise—in the above article. Working with such inspiration, I'll now provide you with a *principle* and a *power question.*

Principle:
Praise is a strong support for people to have the energy to achieve more.

Power Question:
How will you keep track of people's praiseworthy efforts and preplan how you will express your appreciation?

* * * * * *

We now turn to this article by Linda Finkle: To communicate well and build good work relationships, it's essential to look at how you are communicating with your tone and more than just your words.

All Aboard the Communication Train
by Linda Finkle

Communication is more than just the words coming out of your mouth. We send messages to people in ways we may not even think of. You must be cognoscente of the things you do, as the people around us are receiving messages through these non-verbal communication clues. I'm sure you've already heard about standing with your arms crossed and how that can make people feel that you are closed off to them; but have you thought about these other forms of non-verbal communication?

For instance, if you are constantly shutting your door to your office, your colleagues may view this as you are not open to communication. What about not speaking at all (silence)? If you are not communicating at all, you may be coming across as disinterested. The same feeling comes from your eyes focusing on someone or something else. Lastly, the tone in your voice, your inflection and/or how quickly you are speaking are all forms of communication outside of the spoken word itself. While we may view these non-verbal ways of communication as barriers, they are merely just factors we need to be aware of when we are trying to communicate with one another.

So what are barriers to communication we might face?

Clearly cultural differences create a barrier that might be hard to overcome. Gender differences, speaking a different language and vocabulary, the actual words themselves can impact how effective our communication is with each other. So what happens when we face one of these barriers? How do we get the conversation "back on track"?

You must first recognize that you are off track. This could possibly be the hardest step in the process. Once you see that your communication has reached a barrier, it is time to follow a few steps.

Step 1: Create a safe environment. If the person(s) you are communicating with feels uncomfortable, it will be almost impossible to return to having an effective conversation.

Step 2: Share with your colleague that you feel you are off track.

Step 3: Don't ignore having this conversation. While you may consider it difficult, navigating these conversations can help to make others feel more comfortable.

Step 4: Go back to the objective(s). This step is pretty self-explanatory.

Step 5: Accept responsibility for what went wrong. You have to understand that even if you feel like it was their filters that caused your communication train to derail, you played a factor too. You have to prepare for these communication barriers and take responsibility for why the communication fails if you are not adequately prepared.

Step 6: Be specific. Now is not the time to "beat around the bush" so to speak. If your train has already derailed, you have to commit to getting it back on track. This means…be specific.

Step 7: Don't blame or throw stones. Frankly, this will get you nowhere—fast! People get defensive when they feel blamed and at that point the conversation is over.

Step 8: Deal with the root of the problem, not the symptom. To tackle this step, you must first understand what I mean by the root of the problem versus the symptom. For instance, if your colleague always takes a long time getting things done, you might assume that the root of the problem is time management for them. Perhaps it is, but maybe it's not. Maybe this is just a symptom of the root problem, which is they actually are being given more work than one person can handle.

Step 9: Watch for signs that you are not handling the conversation well. Does the person appear to be defensive? Do they not seem to understand? Are they talking about something completely unrelated? These, among many more, are signs that you might need to re-think what you are saying.

Step 10: It's not what you say, it's how you say it. I know you've heard this before. This relates to the inflection we discussed earlier. A whole lot of communication is received in the tone of voice, words used and body language we use when saying it. Saying "I understand" means something entirely different if your arms are crossed and it's spoken with an attitude in your voice than it would if you looked a person in the eye and sounded sincere. In all relationships, communication is very much dependent on so many moving factors. You must be careful about how you come across to someone. There's another example of those non-verbal communication ques.

George Bernard Shaw said "the single biggest problem in communication is the illusion that it has taken place". I will second that. As I have tried to explain here, there are many factors that might leave us feeling like we communicated one message, while the receiver got something completely different. Does this mean we still communicated? They left with a message right? But was it the message you intended for them to leave with? Communication is a complex formula that changes per situation and for each person we talk with; but once we learn the basics we can factor this formula into any conversation. Happy communicating!

Linda Finkle has 30 years of diverse experience, working with business owners and organizations as a business consultant, executive coach, and advisor. Finkle is a Master Certified Coach through the ICF. As CEO of her organizational coaching firm, Incedo Group, Linda has helped countless companies and professionals nationwide to build internal communication strategies and conflict resolution approaches.

Reach Linda through www.incedogroup.com

We learned about how crucial it is to focus on *how you say things* to insure good, productive communication. With this as inspiration, I'll now provide you with a *principle* and *power questions*.

Principle:
Creating good communication requires you to observe carefully your tone, intentions and body language.

Power Questions:
Are you paying close attention to various factors of communication including your tone? Do you provide a safe environment for communicating? What can you do to improve how you communicate?

A FINAL WORD AND
THE SPRINGBOARD TO YOUR DREAMS

Congratulations on your efforts with this book. Thank you for your attention. When you return to these pages again and again, you can *reenergize yourself.* You will get more value each time you review the steps covered in this book.

If you visit San Francisco, I hope you have the opportunity to be good to your body by walking and enjoying the local sights.

To gain more value and use this book as a springboard, be sure to go through it and note your new tasks *in your calendar.* Take some action. Any action towards improving skills and enlarging your life is helpful. I often say, "Better than zero."

* * *

Please consider gaining special training through my coaching (phone and in-person). **I serve as an Executive Coach and Spoken Word Strategist** for people rising in companies, CEOs, business owners, and others seeking to fulfill Big Dreams. I also train people through my keynote presentations, workshops, and Top Five Group Elite Video Training.

My popular **keynote speech is: The 3 C's of Success: Charisma, Confidence and Control of Time.**

My coaching features innovations: *Dynamic Rehearsal* and *Power Rehearsal for Crisis.* Due to my background in improvisation and training in acting, directing and screenwriting, I help clients *as I improvise dialogue* during rehearsal sessions. I coach clients to prepare for speeches and any tough or vital conversation with audiences, colleagues, sales prospects and even family members.

As you continue to work toward expanding your financial abundance and fulfillment in life, you are likely to come up against some tough situations. To be supportive I've written 27 books including . . .

- *Darkest Secrets of Charisma*
- *Be Heard and Be Trusted*
- *Darkest Secrets of Persuasion and Seduction Masters: How to Protect Yourself and Turn the Power to Good*
- *Darkest Secrets of Negotiation Masters*
- *Darkest Secrets of Making a Pitch to the Film and Television Industry*
- *Darkest Secrets of Film Directing*
- *Now You See Me: Make Great First Impressions ... Power Networking*
- *Success Secrets of Rich, Smart and Powerful People: How You Can Use Leverage for Business Success*

See my blog at
www.BeHeardandBeTrusted.com

The best to you,
Tom
Tom Marcoux,
CEO
Executive Coach
Spoken Word Strategist
America's Communication Coach, TFG Thought Leader,
Motion Picture Director, Actor, Producer, Screenwriter

P.S. See **Free Chapters** of Tom Marcoux's 27 books
at http://amzn.to/ZiCTRj   (at Amazon.com)

Titles include:
Be Heard and Be Trusted
Nothing Can Stop You This Year!
Truth No One Will Tell You
Yes! Secrets for Your Best Life . . . Law of Attraction . . .
Reduce Clutter, Enlarge Your Life
Power Time Management   — and more.
(For coaching, reach Tom Marcoux
 at tomsupercoach@gmail.com)

EXCERPT FROM

DARKEST SECRETS OF PERSUASION AND SEDUCTION MASTERS: HOW TO PROTECT YOURSELF AND TURN THE POWER TO GOOD

by Tom Marcoux, America's Communication Coach
Copyright Tom Marcoux

. . . Now, I am in my 40's, with gray in my hair, and for 27 years I have been taking action to protect people.

And now is the time for me to protect you with the Countermeasures I reveal in this book.

Every human being needs to be able to
break the trance that a Manipulator creates.
You need to make good decisions
so you are safe and you keep growing
—and you are not cut down and crippled.

This Darkest Secrets material is so intense that I first released it only with the counterbalance of my most energizing and uplifting books, *Nothing Can Stop You This Year!* and *10 Seconds to Wealth: Master the Moment Using Your Divine Gifts.*

An interviewer asked me: "Who can be the Manipulator?"

A co-worker, a boss, a salesperson, someone you're dating, and someone you think is a friend.

Now is the time—this very minute—for me to write this book to protect you.

I must speak the truth.

These Darkest Secrets of "persuasion masters" are ...

Wait a minute! Let's say it plainly: These are the Darkest Secrets of masters of manipulation. Throughout this book, I will call these people what they are: Manipulators.

Dictionary.com defines "manipulate" as "To influence or manage shrewdly or deviously.... To tamper with or falsify for personal gain."

In this book, we will look on a manipulator as one who deviously influences someone with no concern about that person's well-being, and who causes harm to that person.

Here is the first Darkest Secret:

Darkest Secret #1:
Manipulators Make You Hurt
and Then Offer the Salve.

Manipulators would invite you to go out in the sun for hours and then sell you the salve to soothe your burns. The problem is that we don't notice that this is what they're doing.

For example, you're considering the purchase of a house. A Manipulator asks the question, "So, where would you put your TV?" This question is designed to put you into a trance.

Dictionary.com defines "trance" as "a half-conscious state, seemingly between sleeping and waking, in which ability to function voluntarily may be suspended." Let's condense this: in a trance you may not be able to function freely.

Here is the second Secret:

Darkest Secret #2:

Manipulators Put You into a Trance.

To protect yourself, you must learn to use Countermeasures to Break the Trance.

All the Countermeasures (actions you can take to break the trance) in this book will make you stronger and more capable of protecting yourself.

Now, we'll view the third Secret:

Darkest Secret #3:

Manipulators Care Nothing for You and Human Decency: They'll lie, cheat, and do whatever they need to do so they win—but their charm masks all this.

Let's return to the example of a Manipulator selling you a house. A Manipulator does not pause for an instant to see if you can truly afford the new house. The Manipulator would neglect to mention that you will not only have your mortgage payment of $900. There will be additional costs: home repairs, property tax, water, electricity, homeowner's insurance, and more. The Manipulator only emphasizes what he or she knows you want to hear: "Look! $900 is better than the $1500 you're paying for rent, which is just going down the toilet. And the $900 is an investment."

Let's go back to **Darkest Secret #1:**

Manipulators make you hurt and then offer the salve.

The Manipulator has you feeling good about the solution (salve) and feeling bad about your current life situation.

How? A Manipulator will make you hurt through questions such as:

• What bothers you about paying $1500 a month for rent? (The Manipulator will use a derisive tone when he says the word rent.)

• What is not smart about paying rent on someone else's house instead of investing in your own house?

• How do you feel about your children walking in the

neighborhood where you live now?

Do you see how these questions are designed to make you hurt enough so that you'll buy?

An interviewer asked me, "Tom, aren't these good arguments for purchasing a house?"

"What we're looking at is the *intention* of the influencer," I replied. "Let's look at our definition of a manipulator as one who deviously influences someone with no concern about that person's well-being, and who causes harm to that person. If the person truly cannot afford the house, he or she will be harmed by buying it. If the manipulator conceals the truth, the manipulator is doing harm. That's the important difference."

Some friends of mine are ethical and helpful real estate agents who truthfully reveal the whole situation and help the purchaser achieve her own goals.

In this book, we are talking about another type of person; that is, unethical Manipulators.

* * *

In any given moment, we need to remember the tactics Manipulators use. We will focus on the word D.A.R.K. so you can remember details easily and protect yourself from Manipulators.

D — Dangle something for nothing

A — Alert to scarcity

R — Reveal the Desperate Hot Button

K — Keep on pushing buttons

1. Dangle Something for Nothing

What do conmen and conwomen do to seize your attention? They make you think you're getting a "steal."

I recently saw a documentary in which a conman on a street in England showed a toy that looked like it was dancing. This fake product was actually dancing because of a hidden, invisible thread. The conman was dangling something for nothing. The Entranced Buyer thought he was getting something worth $20 for only $5. That was the trick. The Entranced Buyer felt that he was getting $15 extra of value for his $5. What the Buyer really got was something worth nothing. Similarly, I know someone who purchased a copy of a Disney movie from a street vendor in San Francisco. She brought the copy home and it was unwatchable—and the street vendor was never seen again.

An old phrase goes, "A conman cannot con someone who is not looking for something for nothing."

How to Protect Yourself from "Dangle Something for Nothing"

Stop! Get on your cell phone and talk through the "deal" with someone you know who thinks clearly. Go home. Think about it. Do some research on the Internet. Listen to your gut feelings. If the salesman or conman is too insistent, get away from that Manipulator. Get quiet. Have a cup of water. Cool down. Break the Trance!

Break the Trance and Identify the Crucial Detail

Earlier, I mentioned that a Manipulator puts you into a trance. An added problem is that we put ourselves into a trance. For example, as you read this, are you thinking about your right toe? Most likely not (unless you stubbed your toe recently). The point is that we only focus on a tiny percentage of what is going on in our life.

Around fifteen years ago, I caused myself trouble because

I put myself into a trance. I discovered that under certain conditions, friendship can make you nearly deaf. Here's how: I was producing a song for a motion picture. A good friend was singing backup in the chorus. Because of our friendship, I wanted him to sound great. I completely missed the Crucial Detail. In this kind of situation, the Crucial Detail is that what truly counts is how the lead singer sounds! I made a song that I could not release. What a waste of time and money! I had put myself into a trance.

In any situation in which the Manipulator is "dangling something for nothing," we often fall into a trance and miss the Crucial Detail. The most important detail is *not* that we're saving money if we order before midnight tonight. What counts is whether the product creates a lasting, crucial benefit in our lives. And is the benefit of the product worth the cost? Some people even program themselves to make mistakes by saying, "I can't pass up a bargain." The bargain is *not* the Crucial Detail.

Secrets to Break the Trance

This is the process of B.R.E.A.K.S. It will help you remember the proven methods to break a trance.

B — Breathe

R — Relax

E — Envision

A — Act on aromas

K — Keep moving

S — Smile

Secret #1: Breathe

Remember Secret #1: Manipulators make you hurt and

then offer the salve. The Manipulator wants to put you into a state of being that fills you with a sense of urgency and anxiety. Oh, no! I'm going to miss the sale!

Stop this highly vulnerable state. Take a deep breath. Do it now. Take a deep breath and let your belly "get fat" by filling it with air. As you breathe out, let your belly deflate. Breathe in through your nose and breathe out through your mouth. This is called belly-breathing. Repeat the actions of belly-breathing three times. Good. Now, do you feel different? Remember, when you are relaxed, you are strong.

End of Excerpt from
DARKEST SECRETS OF PERSUASION AND SEDUCTION MASTERS: HOW TO PROTECT YOURSELF AND TURN THE POWER TO GOOD
Copyright Tom Marcoux Media, LLC

Purchase your copy of this book (paperback or ebook) at Amazon.com or BarnesandNoble.com
See **Free Chapters** of Tom Marcoux's 27 books
at http://amzn.to/ZiCTRj

ABOUT THE AUTHOR

Tom Marcoux helps people like you fulfill big dreams. Known as an **Executive Coach - Spoken Word Strategist** and TFG Thought Leader, Tom has authored 27 books with sales in 15 countries. One of his *Darkest Secrets* books rose to #1 on Amazon.com Hot New Releases in Business Life (and in Business Communication). He guides clients and audiences (IBM, Sun Microsystems, etc.) to success in job interviewing, public speaking, media relations, and branding. A member of the National Speakers Association, he is a professional coach and guest expert on TV, radio, and print, and was dubbed "the Personal Branding Instructor" by the *San Francisco Examiner*.

Tom addressed National Association of Broadcasters' Conference six years running. With a degree in psychology, Tom is a guest lecturer at **Stanford University**, DeAnza, & California State University, and teaches business communication, designing careers, public speaking, science fiction cinema/literature and comparative religion at Academy of Art University. Winner of a special award at the **Emmys**, Tom wrote, directed, and produced a feature film that the distributor took to the **Cannes film market**, and the film gained international distribution. He is engaged in book/film projects *Crystal Pegasus* (children's) and *TimePulse* (science fiction). See TomSuperCoach.com and Tom's well-received blog
at www.BeHeardandBeTrusted.com

Consider engaging **Tom Marcoux as your Executive Coach.**

"As Tom's client for many years, I have benefited from

his wisdom and strategic approach. Do your career and personal life a big favor and get his books and engage him as **your Executive Coach**." – Dr. JoAnn Dahlkoetter, author, Your Performing Edge and to CEOs & Olympic Gold Medalists

Tom Marcoux can help you with **speech writing** and **coaching for your best performance.**

As Tom says, *Make Your Speech a Pleasant Beach.*

Join Tom's Linkedin.com group: *Executive Public Speaking and Communication Power.*

At Google+: join the community "Create Your Best Life – Charisma & Confidence"

Get a **Free** report: "9 Deadly Mistakes to Avoid for Your Next Speech and 9 Surefire Methods" at

http://tomsupercoach.com/freereport9Mistakes4Speech.html

Tom Marcoux has trained CEOs, small business owners, and graduate students to speak with impact and gain audiences' tremendous approval and cooperation. *Learn how to present and get thunderous applause!*

"Tom, Thanks for your coaching and work with me on revising my speech at a major university. Working with you has been so enlightening for me. Through your gentle prodding and guidance I was able to write a speech that connects with the audience. I wish everyone could experience the transformation I have undergone. You have helped me discover the warm and compelling stories that now make my speech reach hearts and uplift minds. This was truly an empowering experience. I cannot thank you enough for your great assistance." — J.S.

"Tom Marcoux has been an NAB Conference favorite [speaker] for six years. And he is very energetic."
– John Marino,
Vice President, National Association of Broadcasters,
Washington, D.C.

"Using just one of Tom Marcoux's methods, I got more done in 2 weeks than in 6 months."
– Jaclyn Freitas, M.A.

Tom's Coaching features innovations:
- Dynamic Rehearsal
- Power Rehearsal for Crisis
- The Charisma Advantage that Saves Time

Become a fan of Tom's graphic novels/feature films:
Fantasy Thriller: *Jack AngelSword*
type "JackAngelSword" at Facebook.com

Science fiction: *TimePulse*
www.facebook.com/timepulsegraphicnovel

Children's Fantasy: *Crystal Pegasus*
www.facebook.com/crystalpegasusandrose

See **Free Chapters** of Tom Marcoux's 27 books
at http://amzn.to/ZiCTRj

Special Offer Just for Readers of this Book:

Contact Tom Marcoux at tomsupercoach@gmail.com for special discounts on books, coaching, workshops and presentations. Just mention your experience with this book.

www.ingramcontent.com/pod-product-compliance
Lightning Source LLC
Chambersburg PA
CBHW072136270326
41931CB00010B/1779